S0-BYV-745

PSYCHOLOGICAL

FACTORS

AFFECTING

MEDICAL

CONDITIONS

PSYCHOLOGICAL

FACTORS

AFFECTING

MEDICAL

CONDITIONS

EDITED BY ALAN STOUDEMIRE, M.D.

Washington, DC   American Psychiatric Press, Inc.   London, England

Note: The authors have worked to ensure that all information in this book concerning drug dosages, schedules, and routes of administration is accurate as of the time of publication and consistent with standards set by the U.S. Food and Drug Administration and the general medical community. As medical research and practice advance, however, therapeutic standards may change. For this reason and because human and mechanical errors sometimes occur, we recommend that readers follow the advice of a physician who is directly involved in their care or the care of a member of their family.

Books published by the American Psychiatric Press, Inc., represent the views and opinions of the individual authors and do not necessarily represent the policies and opinions of the Press or the American Psychiatric Association.

Copyright © 1995 American Psychiatric Press, Inc.
ALL RIGHTS RESERVED
Manufactured in the United States of America on acid-free paper
98 97 96 95   4 3 2 1
First Edition

American Psychiatric Press, Inc.
1400 K Street, N.W., Washington, DC   20005

Library of Congress Cataloging-in-Publication Data
Psychological factors affecting medical conditions / edited by Alan
  Stoudemire
      p.   cm.
  Includes bibliographical references and index.
  ISBN 0-88048-708-9 (alk. paper)
  1. Medicine, Psychosomatic.   I. Stoudemire, Alan.
  [DNLM: Disease—psychology.   2. Psychophysiologic
  Disorders.
  WM 90 P97146   1995]
  RC49.P733   1995
  616′.001′9—dc20
  DNLM/DLC
  for Library of Congress   94-27559
                                                                      CIP

British Library Cataloguing in Publication Data
A CIP record is available from the British Library.

Contents

Contributors

Gale Beardsley, M.D.
Clinical Assistant Professor, Department of Psychiatry and Human Behavior, Brown University, Providence, Rhode Island

Claudia Bemis, M.D.
Assistant Professor of Psychiatry, Yale University School of Medicine, New Haven, Connecticut

David G. Folks, M.D.
Professor and Chair, Department of Psychiatry, Creighton-Nebraska Universities, Omaha, Nebraska

Susan Glocheski, M.D.
Clinical Faculty, Department of Psychiatry, Medical College of Virginia, Richmond, Virginia

Michael G. Goldstein, M.D.
Associate Professor of Psychiatry and Human Behavior, Brown University, Providence, Rhode Island

Robert E. Hales, M.D.
Chair, Department of Psychiatry, California Pacific Medical Center, and Clinical Professor, University of California—San Francisco, San Francisco, California

F. Cleveland Kinney, M.D., Ph.D.
Assistant Professor of Psychiatry, University of Alabama, Birmingham, Alabama

James L. Levenson, M.D.
Professor of Psychiatry, Medicine and Surgery, Medical College of Virginia, Richmond, Virginia

M. Eileen McNamara, M.D.
Assistant Professor of Psychiatry and Human Behavior, Brown University, Providence, Rhode Island

Michael G. Moran, M.D.
Associate Professor, University of Colorado School of Medicine and National Jewish Center for Immunology and Respiratory Medicine, Denver, Colorado

Raymond Niaura, Ph.D.
Associate Professor of Psychiatry and Human Behavior, Brown University, Providence, Rhode Island

David Spiegel, M.D.
Professor, Department of Psychiatry and Behavioral Sciences, Stanford University School of Medicine, Stanford, California

Alan Stoudemire, M.D.
Professor, Department of Psychiatry and Behavioral Sciences, Emory University School of Medicine, Atlanta, Georgia

Foreword

Reminding the Body

The mind-body problem is one of the most exciting areas in psychiatric medicine, in part because it has been so long neglected and in part because increasing sophistication in research, methodology, and techniques has made it possible to examine the elegant interrelationships between mind and body. We struggle toward the end of the 20th century with a remarkable array of sophisticated medical techniques ranging from magnetic resonance imaging and positron-emission tomography to studies of neurotransmitter function to genetics, with a 19th century mechanistic view of how the body works. It would be a strange lapse in design indeed if a creature endowed with the unusual proportion of cortex to body mass observed in *Homo sapiens* made little or no use of this cognitive ability in a way that had adaptive value. Similarly, given our human ability to experience, remember, and plan, it would be surprising if adverse social, physical, and psychological events had no affect on the functioning of the body that the mind controls.

Despite this, the systematic study of mind-body interrelationships has received short shrift from medicine because these intangibles were always considered suspect at best, and from psychiatry as well because they did not uniformly involve the study of major psychiatric disorders. Assembled here is an excellent, thoughtful, and scholarly examination of the evidence for and against a relationship between psychological and medical factors, and the onset, course, and treatment of medical conditions. In these reviews, organized by disease and organ system, the authors carefully examine evidence suggesting that psychiatric disorders may complicate medical illness, that personality styles may influence the onset and course of disease, and that psychosocial treatments may influence medical as well as psychiatric outcome. The book moves us forward in consolidating what is known and highlighting clearly what is unknown.

In some cases, constraints are put on generally accepted wisdom. For example, the well-known Type A personality pattern seems to have its best predictive value in general populations rather than in those with coronary disease, suggesting that the relationship is one affecting those at the border between normal and pathological cardiac conditions. Certain aspects of the Type A personality, such as hostility, seem to be the most important. Evidence for a personality style affecting the onset or course of cancer is less clear, although some studies seem to show that a fighting spirit may be associated with a better outcome. The pitfalls of these personality studies are critically examined because there is always the danger of attributing etiologic importance to certain personality factors that are likely to be complications rather than causes of a disease.

The authors in this volume also review a growing body of studies indicating that psychosocial interventions have tangible medical results in helping patients with cardiovascular disease and cancer, in some cases resulting in reduced mortality. The literature on successful psychosocial intervention for other disorders—for example, involving the gastrointestinal, dermatologic, and respiratory systems—is also touched on. These literatures are important not only because they provide guidelines for the acceptance or rejection of new treatments, but also because they turn the theoretically interesting problem—how does the mind influence the body—into a clinically practical one—how can we help patients with medical illnesses to cope with them. As Drs. Stoudemire and Hales note in their excellent overview, the very term *psychological factors affecting physical* (now *medical*) *condition* is awkward, and the category has been underutilized. Nonetheless, the Task Force on DSM-IV wisely decided to include it again in DSM-IV. This diagnostic category pushes us as no other psychiatric diagnosis does to examine systematically the relationship between mind and body and the effects of stress, coping, and psychotherapy on disease incidence and course.

At this relatively youthful stage of its development, this new field of psychosomatic medicine (for want of a better term) raises more questions than it does answers, but they are important questions. What answers we have point toward a fascinating and developing field of psychiatric medicine. Disciplines such as psychoneuroimmunology and psychoneuroendocrinology were virtually unheard of 20 years ago and were hardly taken seriously 10 years ago. They are now flourishing and growing areas providing us with systematic means of examining mechanisms by which psychosocial events may have physiological consequences. "Mens sana in corpore sano" is the old adage. This book reminds us that a sound body may be, in part, the product if not the home of the sound mind.

David Spiegel, M.D.

Introduction

In the process of preparing the fourth edition of the *Diagnostic and Statistical Manual of Mental Disorders* (DSM-IV), extensive background papers were prepared to assess critically the literature for each given diagnostic category. Any proposed changes in DSM-III-R criteria for DSM-IV were to be justified and supported by the research literature. The chapters in this volume were written as part of that process in considering revisions in the DSM-III-R diagnostic category "Psychological Factors Affecting Physical Conditions" (PFAPC) and originally appeared as a series of journal articles in *Psychosomatics*. These articles now appear here in a revised and updated form.

The literature review mandated by the DSM-IV revision process, however, presented a challenge for the group charged with evaluating the category PFAPC. First, the literature regarding the effects of psychological factors, psychiatric disorders, and other behaviors affecting physical conditions was extensive and dated to the early part of this century. Second, there was almost no research using the diagnostic category PFAPC itself, which, although originally appearing as part of DSM-III in 1980, had found essentially no usefulness as a descriptive diagnosis suitable for systematic investigations. Third, the literature that had to be examined was extremely broad and embraced a variety of theoretical fields and clinical disciplines, including traditional psychosomatic medicine, behavioral medicine, health psychology, psychophysiology, and consultation-liaison psychiatry.

Efforts to organize and analyze this vast literature were simplified by several strategies. The primary strategy was to examine primarily studies that had utilized some form of systematic research methodology, which eliminated much of the theoretical and anecdotal literature. Second, rather than focusing on psychophysiologic symptom formation, emphasis was placed on the possible influence of psychological factors and psychiatric disorders on the onset and exacerbation of specific medical disorders. Finally, the literature reviews were primarily divided along the lines of organ systems (e.g., cardiovascular, pulmonary, gastroenterology) as a practical maneuver to divide up the work assignments. These strategies resulted in a series of succinct reviews that identified the scientific evidence for the effects of psychological factors and psychiatric disorders on the onset and exacerbation of medical conditions, including the role of behavioral factors that affect the prognosis of medical disorders. This ambitious project resulted in substantive changes in the DSM-III-R category PFAPC for DSM-IV, which has now been renamed "Psychological Factors Affecting Medical Conditions." Further details for the rationale for these changes, as well as the new diagnostic criteria, are elucidated in the introductory chapter of the volume.

The process could not have been achieved without the hard work and dedication of members of the committee involved in the revision process and the associated authors of the literature reviews. I am greatly indebted to each of these individuals, without whose effort and valuable contributions this volume could not have been completed. It is hoped that as a result of these efforts not only will the new DSM-IV category be more useful for both clinicians and researchers, but also the medical and psychiatric community will have available a scientifically rigorous compendium that documents beyond question the critical role that psychological and psychiatric factors play in the course and outcome of medical illness.

Alan Stoudemire, M.D.

Acknowledgments

I thank the authors of these literature reviews, members of the DSM-IV Work Group examining Psychological Factors Affecting Physical Conditions, and the many consultants who contributed to the process. Special thanks are also due to Dr. Robert Hales for his excellent guidance and support in his role as Chair of the Psychiatric Systems Interface Disorders, the parent committee for our work group's activities, and to Dr. Michael First for his help in refining the diagnostic criteria. Special thanks are also extended to Dr. Allen Frances for his vision and leadership in bringing the DSM-IV process to a successful conclusion. Finally, the outstanding efforts of Ms. Lynda Mathews, my administrative assistant at Emory University School of Medicine, are also recognized. Without her help and tireless dedication, this and many other projects would never have been brought to realization.

Members of the DSM-IV Psychological Factors Affecting Physical Conditions Work Group

Alan Stoudemire, M.D. (Chair)
Gale Beardsley, M.D.
David G. Folks, M.D.
Michael G. Goldstein, M.D.

James L. Levenson, M.D.
M. Eileen McNamara, M.D.
Michael G. Moran, M.D.
Raymond Niaura, Ph.D.

Consultants to the Work Group

Arthur J. Barsky, M.D.
Jimmie C. Holland, M.D.
Roger Kathol, M.D.
Donald S. Kornfeld, M.D.
Z. J. Lipowski, M.D.
Don R. Lipsitt, M.D.

George B. Murray, M.D.
Perry M. Nicassio, Ph.D.
Robert O. Pasnau, M.D.
Samuel W. Perry III, M.D.
Troy L. Thompson II, M.D.
Thomas N. Wise, M.D.

CHAPTER 1

Psychological Factors Affecting Medical Conditions and DSM-IV

An Overview

ALAN STOUDEMIRE, M.D.
ROBERT E. HALES, M.D.

The belief that psychological factors influence the expression of physical symptoms and may affect the course of medical illness has been a basic assumption inherent in the practice of medicine since the time of Hippocrates. The scientific traditions of 20th-century psychosomatic theory and research that have supported this belief represent a variety of disciplines and theoretical perspectives (Alexander 1950; Beaumont 1833; Cannon 1915; Cassel 1976; Dunbar 1935; Meyer 1957; Pavlov 1902; Selye 1946; Wolff 1953). The major trends in the field of modern "psychosomatic medicine" derive from three major designated areas of theory and scientific investigation: psychoanalysis, psychophysiology, and psychobiology (Lipowski 1986a). Each of these major areas is briefly considered as they have contributed to this field of study.

The psychoanalytic tradition in psychosomatic medicine was most prominently represented by Franz Alexander (1950) and his now discarded "specificity theory." Although Alexander foresaw and advocated a multifactorial model of illness in which psychological factors interacted with biological, environmental, and social influences, the field of psychosomatic medicine has as yet to recover fully from the misconceptions that arose from the belief that specific constellations of intrapsychic conflicts resulted in specific types of physical illness. The tradition respectfully survives, however, in a modified form in the research on Type A behavior in which elements of hostility are now proposed to be the specific cardio-toxic component of the Type A personality style that accelerates athero-sclerosis. Heightened physiologic reactivity in such individuals, resulting in acute and chronic activation of the sympathetic nervous systems, is one mechanism in which atherosclerosis and cardiac arrhythmias are more likely to develop. Although largely passé in their original theoretical for-mulations, psychoanalytic theories of psychosomatic illness served to stimulate scientific interest and research into the relationships between behavior and disease processes.

The psychophysiologic tradition in psychosomatic research derives from the classic studies of Pavlov (1902) and Cannon (1915) and was systematically elaborated by Harold G. Wolff (1953), who eloquently set forth psychosocial concepts of stressful life events as precipitators of dis-ease. As Lipowski observed (1986a), Wolff's emphasis on controlled sci-entific methodological techniques to measure the relationship between stressful stimuli and physiologic variables set the technical standards for subsequent modern psychophysiologic studies in psychoneurophysiol-ogy, psychoneuroendocrinology, and psychoneuroimmunology.

The so-called psychobiological model is represented by the work of Adolph Meyer (1957), who was one of the most influential American psychiatrists in the first half of this century. Meyer's theories involved utilizing comprehensive patient assessments to arrive at case formula-tions in an attempt to understand the interactions among constitutional, environmental, and developmental factors for each given patient (Meyer 1957). This psychobiological perspective, from which the now popular-ized "biopsychosocial" model is a derivative, was influential in the sub-sequent work of a disciple of Meyer, Helen Flanders Dunbar (1935), who was the primary organizational founder of the psychosomatic medicine movement in the United States (Lipowski 1986a). As noted by Lipowski, the psychobiological approach of Meyer and Dunbar formed the primary theoretical basis for clinical and epidemiologic studies that attempted to ascertain relationships between social factors and personality character-istics, with vulnerability to disease. Mainstream psychosomatic medicine research (cardiovascular psychophysiology, psychoneuroendocrinology, and psychoneuroimmunology) is based on this tradition (Lipowski 1986a).

More recently, particularly as a result of the growth of consultation-liaison psychiatry, the adverse effect of psychiatric disorders (such as depression and delirium) on medical outcome in hospitalized patients has been examined (Guze and Daengsurisri 1967; Hale et al. 1977), and the beneficial effects of psychiatric consultation and treatment of similar patients has been documented (Cassem and Hackett 1983). These clinical studies supplement epidemiologic reports that have found, for example, increased rates of medical morbidity in medical outpatients who are depressed (Carney et al. 1988).

A significant body of data, much of it derived from the Medical Outcomes Study funded by the Rand Corporation, has supported the fact that depression is associated with as much limitation in daily functioning and well-being as are most common medical conditions (Wells and Burnam 1991). Other data, derived from primary care settings, also have supported the observation that patients with major depression have more physical illness than nondepressed patients and that somatic symptoms of major depression exacerbate the functional disability associated with physical illness (Coulehan et al. 1990). In psychiatric illness, patients with comorbid medical conditions have increased chronicity and lower recovery rates as compared with depressed patients without concurrent medical illness (Keitner et al. 1991).

In a group of 211 medical patients with life-threatening illnesses (myocardial infarction, subarachnoid hemorrhage, acute upper gastrointestinal hemorrhage, and pulmonary embolism) who were evaluated once they had stabilized, the presence of depression in the recovery period predicted a much poorer outcome in the first month following their admission. Of the patients with depression, 47% either died or had subsequent life-threatening complications as compared with 10% for similar complications in the nondepressed patients (Silverstone 1990). Clinical depression also complicates and negatively affects outcome in stroke patients. Clinical depression occurring after stroke has been well documented to impair recovery from stroke and has a negative impact on recovery in functional status and cognitive performance (Morris et al. 1992). Depressed patients with a history of myocardial infarction have a particularly poor clinical prognosis and a higher rate of chronicity in their depressive symptoms as compared with medical patients without a history of myocardial infarction (Wells et al. 1993). Major depression in patients hospitalized after a myocardial infarction has been shown to be an independent risk factor for mortality. The presence of major depression following a myocardial infarction contributes to increased subsequent mortality at least as much as does left ventricular failure and a previous history of myocardial infarction (Frasure-Smith et al. 1993). Improved psychosocial adjustment (Evans et al. 1988) and survival (Spiegel et al. 1989) are possible when timely psychiatric intervention is instituted in the context of combined medical and psychiatric illness. For example, it has been demonstrated that psychiatric interventions that enhance effective coping and reduce affective distress have beneficial effects on long-term survival in both breast cancer patients and patients with malignant melanoma (Fawzy et al. 1993; Spiegel et al. 1989).

It is now generally accepted that the relationship between psychological factors and medical conditions is complex and may be affected by numerous biological and psychosocial variables. Measuring interactive effects between these multiple factors and evaluating the variability of their biological influence on the individual are the major challenges facing researchers today. For example, if so-called Type A behavior carries a true risk for the development of coronary artery disease (Rosenman et al. 1975), many other variables that might affect outcome in any given individual must be controlled to measure the contribution of such a psychological or behavioral factor, such as genetic factors, diet, exercise, smoking, presence or absence of other coexistent confounding stresses (e.g., marital, financial, legal), occupational exposure risks, and the presence or absence of concurrent medical or psychiatric illness. The difficulty of controlling these multiple interacting variables may at least partially explain the variability of findings in the area (Dimsdale 1988).

Even the effects of "stress," a fundamental component of psychosomatic theory, have proven to be complex and problematic to measure. Often mistakenly considered to be deleterious in and of itself, stress may have beneficial, negative, or mixed effects on the individual. For example, Selye described "eustress" and "distress," the first facilitating growth and healing, and the latter precipitating disease. Moreover, whether or not a given event will be (negatively) stressful for an individual depends on the personalized meaning of the event to the individual (the "cognitive appraisal" of the event or situation) and the abilities of the individual to manage, adapt, or "cope" with the stress at hand (Lazarus 1966). In addition, evidence exists that vulnerability and resistance to stress may be affected by the relative presence or absence of social "buffers" that may impart protection against emotional disequilibrium and physical illness. Even the classic work of Holmes and Rahe (1967), which popularized the potential deleterious "life-change" effects on the onset of physical illness, was criticized, because in evaluating the effects of life change, the personalized meaning of life events for the individual must be considered in the process (Craig and Brown 1984).

Increased emphasis has been placed on epidemiologic research that has identified characteristics that form "risk factors" for the development of physical illness. This research has documented such behavioral factors as cigarette smoking, obesity, alcohol and substance dependency, and unsafe sexual practices as major contributors to premature death and unnecessary medical morbidity in the United States, much of it theoretically preventable (Stoudemire et al. 1987a). For example, the total number of annual premature deaths in the United States (excluding acquired immunodeficiency syndrome [AIDS]) was almost 2 million based on 1980 population data. One may also add to these figures approximately 26,000 deaths per year from suicide (Amler and Eddins 1987; Stoudemire et al. 1987b) (Table 1–1 and Figure 1–1).

Although it can be seen from Table 1–1 that behaviorally related effects have a major impact on the public health in the United States and that the evidence for these effects is incontrovertible, factors that contribute to the majority of this morbidity and mortality—such as cigarette smoking, obesity, and alcoholism—have customarily received relatively little attention in both general psychiatry and traditional psychosomatic medicine.

In Table 1–2 we outlined a scheme (modeled in part after a format used by Lipowski [1986b]) for classifying the areas in which psychological, behavioral, and social factors may affect physical health. Section I embraces most of what has been traditionally subsumed under the rubric of psychosomatic medicine. Behavioral physiology would include the study of gross pathophysiologic reactions to various psychosocial factors and experimental stress paradigms, as well as investigation of their bio-

TABLE 1–1.　Major precursors of premature death, United States, 1980: attributable deaths, years lost before age 65, and days of hospital care

Precursor	Deaths	Potential years lost before age 65	Days of hospital care
Tobacco	338.022	1,497.161	16,098.587
High blood pressure	297.162	340.752	9,781.647
Overnutrition (obesity, dietary factors)	289.502	292.960	16,306.194
Alcohol total	99.247	1,795.458	3,348.354
Injury	53.683	1,497.206	2,229.824
Other	45.564	298.252	1,118.530
Injury risks (excluding alcohol)	64.169	1,755.720	25,470.176
Gaps in screening	56.592	172.793	3,647.729
Gaps in primary prevention	54.027	1,273.631	4,651.730
Inadequate access to care	21.974	324.709	2,141.569
Occupation	16.807	102.065	581.740
Handguns	13.365	350.683	28.514
Unintended pregnancy	8.000	520.000	NA
Total preventable	1,258.867	8,425.932	82,056.240
(percentage)	(63.1)	(70.8)	(29.9)
Total all causes	1,995.000	11,897.174	274,508.000

Source.　Reprinted from Amler RW, Eddins DL: "Cross-Sectional Analysis: Precursors of Premature Death in the United States." *American Journal of Preventive Medicine* 3 (suppl 5):181–187, 1987, p. 184. Used with permission.

chemical regulation. Section II covers the effects of formally defined psychiatric disorders on the course of medical illness, a subject that has been of major interest to consultation-liaison psychiatrists. Section III includes the major public health concerns of behavior noted earlier that comprise major "risk factors" for a variety of illnesses, including cardiovascular disease, cancer, and AIDS, as well as individual and group effects of life change associated with illness vulnerability.

As may be seen from this format, the behavioral and psychological factors that may affect medical health are broader than what has traditionally been considered the general boundaries of psychosomatic medicine and psychophysiology. The categorization scheme allows for the incorporation of many of the public health factors that have such a major im-

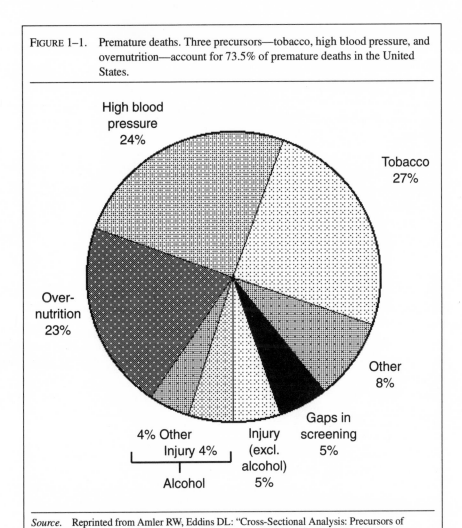

FIGURE 1–1.   Premature deaths. Three precursors—tobacco, high blood pressure, and overnutrition—account for 73.5% of premature deaths in the United States.

High blood pressure 24%

Tobacco 27%

Over-nutrition 23%

Other 8%

4% Other

Injury 4%

Alcohol

Injury (excl. alcohol) 5%

Gaps in screening 5%

Source.   Reprinted from Amler RW, Eddins DL: "Cross-Sectional Analysis: Precursors of Premature Death in the United States." *American Journal of Preventive Medicine* 3 (suppl 5):181–187, 1987, p. 185. Used with permission.

pact on the American population, as well as of the effects of comorbid psychiatric illness on medical outcome. It may be readily seen, therefore, that any diagnostic or categorization classification used to address the traditional concern of psychosomatic medicine should address these issues. It is with these considerations that the DSM-III-R (American Psychiatric Association 1987) category Psychological Factors Affecting Physical Condition (PFAPC) was reevaluated for possible revisions in

TABLE 1–2. Psychological and behavioral factors affecting medical conditions

I. Behavioral physiology (psychophysiology)
 A. Physiological reactions to psychological and behavioral variables
 B. Biological regulatory mechanisms associated with behavioral and psychological variables
  1. Psychoneurophysiology
  2. Psychoneuroendocrinology
  3. Psychoneuroimmunology
  4. Cardiovascular psychophysiology
II. Effects of concurrent psychiatric illness on the course and outcome of medical disorders
III. Behavioral risk factors for disease and injury
 A. Personality variables
 B. Cigarette smoking
 C. Dietary habits
 D. Alcohol and substance abuse
 E. Hazardous sexual behavior
 F. Risk-taking behaviors (accidents, injury)
 G. Noncompliance with medical treatment
 H. Violence, suicide, homicide
 I. Stressful or disruptive life change

Source. Modeled in part after Lipowski 1986b.

DSM-IV (American Psychiatric Association 1994); the process of that review is the focus of the latter part of this chapter.

PFAPC and DSM-IV

Despite the complexities in ascertaining precise associations among psychological and behavioral factors and medical conditions, a reasonable amount of empirically based evidence now exists to affirm beyond any reasonable doubt that psychological factors do affect physical health and the onset and outcome of at least some medical illnesses. Various issues—including the precise types of psychological and behavioral "factors" that are involved, the types of individuals who are susceptible to them, the specific types of illnesses in which such effects are important, and at what point during the course of a physical illness they are primarily operative—remain unresolved.

From a diagnostic standpoint, these effects were recognized in DSM-II (American Psychiatric Association 1968) primarily under the rubric of "psychophysiologic" disorders. In DSM-III (American Psychiatric Association 1980) a substantial change in terminology occurred in which the category PFAPC was adopted.

In DSM-III, PFAPC was primarily based on a background paper in which Looney and colleagues (1978) proposed abandoning the DSM-II term *psychophysiologic*. This argument was based on eight major points: 1) the DSM-II term *psychophysiologic* was rarely used as a diagnosis; 2) the decision as to whether a patient's condition was psychophysiologic or organic was arbitrary; 3) the term was believed to decrease collaboration among specialists; 4) the term perpetuated simplistic ideas about disease etiology; 5) the term was often used as a "last resort" when previous efforts at medical diagnosis and treatment had failed; 6) the term was deficient because it referred only to causation and did not address how psychosocial factors might perpetuate or exacerbate a physical problem; 7) no clear operational criteria were defined; and 8) the DSM-II classification of psychophysiologic disorders was inadequate for methodological research purposes.

The DSM-III PFAPC category that was proposed and subsequently adopted was believed to offer significant advantages over the DSM-II psychophysiologic terminology because it integrated psychological contributions to medical illness into a multiaxial diagnostic system. PFAPC, however, was always considered to be a "category" and not a diagnosis per se. PFAPC represented a "diagnosis modifier rather than a psychological diagnosis as a separate entity" (Looney et al. 1978, p. 307). The intent was "to provide the clinician with a marker or label that would focus attention on clinically important information but not mislead anyone into thinking that a given condition need be considered either psychological or organic" (Looney et al. 1978, p. 307). Hence, if a clinician believed that psychological factors were significant in the patient's condition, this observation could be noted on Axis I by denoting PFAPC, with the physical disorder on Axis III then noted. By enlarging the scope from the DSM-II psychophysiologic disorders, it was hoped that in DSM-III the new category and the multiaxial system would broaden the range of psychological and behavioral factors considered to contribute to the onset or exacerbation of physical illnesses (Linn and Spitzer 1982).

Despite this rationale and the ultimate adoption of the conceptual framework of the PFAPC category in the DSM-III nomenclature, there is little evidence to suggest that the category PFAPC had any greater success than its DSM-II "psychophysiologic" predecessor. Despite a considerable upsurge in interest in psychosocial and behavioral factors in the etiology and course of physical disorders—and progressive improvement in the quality of research in this area—almost no research in either the medical or psychiatric literature using this term has been generated (Popkin 1987). Fewer than 10 articles have ever been published that use the term "PFAPC" in their title or as a substantial component of their content; no articles were found that use it as a basis for empirical research.

In his exhaustive review of the development of DSM-III and DSM-III-R, Skodol (1989) noted the apparent failure of the PFAPC category to achieve clinical or research use.

> PFAPC has not lived up to the expectations held for it with respect to stimulating dialogue between psychiatrists and nonpsychiatric physicians [Skodol citing Mezzich 1987]. There have been no studies to date of use of the diagnosis; and from consultation-liaison services where the diagnosis would be expected to be used most frequently, problems with its use have been reported. (p. 325)

Skodol also discussed the problem inherent in this category of what constitutes "psychological factors":

> In DSM-III, something "psychological" was referred to as "the meaning ascribed to environmental stimuli by the individual" [Skodol quoting DSM-III, p. 303]. Examples given were stimuli arising from interpersonal relations, such as arguments or the loss of a loved one. The person himself or herself may or may not be aware of the meaning he or she ascribes to the stimuli, or of the relationship of the stimuli to the initiation or exacerbation of the physical condition. When a judgment of such a high order of inference is involved in determining that psychological factors may be present, one might expect considerable unreliability in the use of the diagnosis. One clinician's interpretation of the meaning ascribed to the event or situation and its role in the illness process could easily conflict with the judgment of a second clinician. (pp. 325–326)

Members of the DSM-IV Work Group charged with developing updated diagnostic criteria for this category attempted to identify problems and to outline options for possible revisions in a series of publications (Stoudemire et al. 1989). The major options that were considered included the following:

1. Allow the category to stand as it is, without significant changes.
2. Discard the category altogether or use other psychiatric diagnoses (such as adjustment disorders) whenever possible in the context of medical illness.
3. Remove the category from the mental disorders section of DSM-IV and include it as a "V Code."
4. Include PFAPC in a special section called "Other Clinically Significant Conditions" to set the category apart from the more formally defined "Mental Disorders" section of DSM-IV.
5. Delete the category as a freestanding entity, but further adapt the existing multiaxial system to designate more clearly adverse relationships between Axis I and Axis III disorders (and vice versa).
6. Structure the criteria more rigorously to allow clinicians the option of subcategorizing the predominant types of "psychological factors" that are considered to be related in the patient's physical illness.

After extensive study of the available literature and analysis of surveys of national experts in psychosomatic medicine, behavioral medicine, consultation-liaison psychiatry, and health psychology, the DSM-IV PFAPC Subcommittee concluded that the consensus was that, problematic as the category was, and despite its lack of use since its conception in DSM-III, the category should be retained and should still be used as a "mainstream" diagnostic entity. To revise the category to make it more clinically useful, a subcategorization format was developed that would allow clinicians to specify the major type of psychological or behavioral factor assessed to be operative in affecting the patient's medical condition; the factors so designated would include the broad range of psychological, social, and behavioral phenomena noted in Table 1–2 that appear to affect physical health. It was believed that the category should be broader, accounting for more than reactions to "environmental stimuli," which was the primary focus of DSM-III and DSM-III-R.

In an effort to identify these types of psychological and behavioral factors for which empiric evidence exists to support such an association, extensive literature reviews were undertaken. The purpose and methodology of these reviews are described below.

Purpose and Methodology of the Literature Reviews

The purpose of the literature reviews were as follows:

1. Document the existing literature that would confirm that psychological factors affect medical illness.
2. Delineate the specific types of psychological and behavioral factors that could affect specific types of medical conditions.
3. Identify at what phase of medical illness evidence exists that psychological factors actually have some effect on the course of a medical illness.
4. Document options and recommendations for new diagnostic criteria for PFAPC in DSM-IV.

Performing comprehensive and critical reviews of the relationships between psychological factors and medical conditions presented a formidable task. A survey of the more recent literature (focusing on empirical studies) was simplified by two strategies. First, work was distributed primarily along an "organ system" basis (cardiology, gastroenterology, endocrine, dermatology, pulmonary, immunology, rheumatology, neurology, oncology, and nephrology). In addition, "life-style risk factors," which focused on cigarette smoking and obesity, were also examined. Attention was focused primarily on studies that employed some degree of systematic data-based methodology (preferably in a controlled fashion) and on those involving collection of empiric data, rather than anecdotal case reports.

Because the effects of certain types of autonomic nervous system arousal are now well accepted and expressed primarily in focal and usually transient single symptoms (sympathetic autonomic symptoms such as palpitations, transient elevations in blood pressure, urinary frequency, diaphoresis, nausea, dyspnea, diarrhea, urinary retention, dizziness), these focal psychophysiologic symptoms were not reviewed in detail. Such symptoms were considered to be extremely common and well described clinically in both the medical and psychiatric literature and were considered in the process of the project only if they were part of sign- and symptom-based medical "syndromes" that had been well defined for systemic study (e.g., irritable bowel syndrome). Moreover, the committee did not attempt a detailed review or critique of basic science psychophysiologic research and its various subcomponents (i.e., neurophysiology, psychoneuroendocrinology, psychoneuroimmunology) unless specific studies apparently confirmed a mediating link between psychological and behavioral variables and well-defined medical disorders. The purpose of this category within the context of a diagnostic manual of clinical psychiatric syndromes was considered by clinicians to define links between such psychological variables and medical illness. Finally, the committee did not undertake a review of social and cultural variables affecting physical illness (i.e., medical sociology) because this was considered beyond the scope of the diagnostic category.

Assuming that the literature reviews would yield reliable data confirming the existence of a spectrum of conditions and provide enough evidence to support the validity of a categorical entity such as PFAPC, the committee sought to identify factors that could facilitate development of more rigorous criteria for the category. The most likely possibility for increasing the rigor of the diagnosis would be, as noted above, to identify specific types of psychological factors that have an effect on physical conditions, supported by reliable data. Because the vagueness and ambiguity of the PFAPC category were two of the reasons most frequently cited by expert clinicians that the designation was rarely used, it was hoped that this would be a reasonable goal from which to begin the literature analysis.

Based on the information collected from the reviews, proposed diagnostic criteria were developed. Shown in Table 1–3 are the final criteria for DSM-IV, which were reviewed and critiqued not only by members of the committee but also by the Psychiatric Systems Interface Disorders Work Group, the DSM-IV Task Force, and distinguished experts from around the country who served as advisers to the committee since 1988, when work was first begun on this project.

All reviews in this volume employed standardized computer-assisted literature searches of the international literature on human research in the area of psychiatric, psychological, and behavioral factors affecting the

TABLE 1–3.   DSM-IV diagnostic criteria for psychological factor affecting medical
            condition

A.   A general medical condition (coded on Axis III) is present.

B.   Psychological factors adversely affect the general medical condition in one of the
     following ways:

    (1)   the factors have influenced the course of the general medical condition as
            shown by a close temporal association between the psychological factors
            and the development or exacerbation of, or delayed recovery from, the
            general medical condition

    (2)   the factors interfere with the treatment of the general medical condition

    (3)   the factors constitute additional health risks for the individual

    (4)   stress-related physiological responses precipitate or exacerbate symptoms of
            the general medical condition

**Choose name based on the nature of the psychological factors (if more than one
factor is present, indicate the most prominent):**

Mental Disorder Affecting . . . *[Indicate the General Medical Condition]* (e.g., an
Axis I disorder such as Major Depressive Disorder delaying recovery from a
myocardial infarction)

Psychological Symptoms Affecting . . . *[Indicate the General Medical Condition]*
(e.g., depressive symptoms delaying recovery from surgery; anxiety exacerbating
asthma)

Personality Traits or Coping Style Affecting . . . *[Indicate the General Medical
Condition]* (e.g., pathological denial of the need for surgery in a patient with
cancer; hostile, pressured behavior contributing to cardiovascular disease)

Maladaptive Health Behaviors Affecting . . . *[Indicate the General Medical
Condition]* (e.g., overeating; lack of exercise; unsafe sex)

Stress-Related Physiological Response Affecting . . . *[Indicate the General Medical
Condition]* (e.g., stress-related exacerbations of ulcer, hypertension, arrhythmia, or
tension headache)

Other or Unspecified Psychological Factors Affecting . . . *[Indicate the General
Medical Condition]* (e.g., interpersonal, cultural, religious factors)

Source.   Reprinted from American Psychiatric Association: *Diagnostic and Statistical Manual
of Mental Disorders,* 4th Edition. Washington, DC, American Psychiatric Association, 1994,
p. 678. Used with permission. Copyright 1994 American Psychiatric Association.

predisposition, onset, exacerbation, perpetuation, maintenance, or relapse of physical illnesses. Specific types of psychological, psychiatric,
and behavioral factors that were researched included formal Axis I and
Axis II DSM-III-R diagnoses, symptoms of anxiety and depression, behavioral patterns and personality factors, and physiologic responses to

environmental or experimental stimuli. Alcoholism and eating disorders were not considered because other DSM-IV committees were evaluating these areas.

This volume provides these reviews, which have undergone additional editing; the references are updated through 1993. This volume considers cardiovascular disease (Chapters 2 and 3), neurological conditions (Chapter 4), cancer (Chapter 5), gastrointestinal conditions (Chapter 6), dermatologic conditions (Chapter 7), pulmonary and rheumatologic diseases (Chapter 8), renal disease (Chapter 9), and endocrine diseases (Chapter 10). It is hoped that this project will facilitate the consolidation of the literature involving possible relationships between psychological factors and medical illness and stimulate a critical reexamination of the strengths and weaknesses of the various research methodologies employed, as well as lead to further research to clarify many remaining areas of uncertainty.

References

Alexander F: Psychosomatic Medicine. New York, WW Norton, 1950

American Psychiatric Association: Diagnostic and Statistical Manual of Mental Disorders, 2nd Edition. Washington, DC, American Psychiatric Association, 1968

American Psychiatric Association: Diagnostic and Statistical Manual of Mental Disorders, 3rd Edition. Washington, DC, American Psychiatric Association, 1980

American Psychiatric Association: Diagnostic and Statistical Manual of Mental Disorders, 3rd Edition, Revised. Washington, DC, American Psychiatric Association, 1987

American Psychiatric Association: Diagnostic and Statistical Manual of Mental Disorders, 4th Edition. Washington, DC, American Psychiatric Association, 1994

Amler RW, Eddins DL: Cross-sectional analysis: precursors of premature death in the United States. American Journal of Preventive Medicine 3 (suppl 5):181–187, 1987

Beaumont W: Experiments and Observations on the Gastric Juice and the Physiology of Digestion. Plattsburg, NY, FP Allen, 1833

Cannon WB: Bodily Changes in Pain, Hunger, Fear, and Rage. New York, Appleton, 1915

Carney RM, Rich MW, Freedland KE: Major depressive disorder predicts cardiac events in patients with coronary artery disease. Psychosom Med 50:627–633, 1988

Cassel J: The contribution of the social environment to host resistance. Am J Epidemiol 104:107–123, 1976

Cassem NH, Hackett TP: Psychiatric consultation in a coronary care unit. Ann Intern Med 75:9–14, 1983

Coulehan JL, Schulberg HC, Block MR, et al: Medical comorbidity of major depressive disorder in a primary medical practice. Arch Intern Med 150:2363–2367, 1990

Craig TKJ, Brown GW: Life events, meaning and physical illness: a review, in Health Care and Human Behavior. Edited by Steptoe A, Matthews A. London, Academic Press, 1984, pp 7–39

Dimsdale JE: Research links between psychiatry and cardiology. Gen Hosp Psychiatry 10:328–338, 1988

Dunbar H: Emotions and Bodily Changes: A Survey of Literature on Psychosomatic Relationships: 1910–1933. New York, Columbia University Press, 1935

Evans DL, McCartney CF, Haggerty JJ, et al: Treatment of depression in cancer patients is associated with better life adaptation: a pilot study. Psychosom Med 50:72–76, 1988

Fawzy FI, Fawzy NW, Hyun CS, et al: Malignant melanoma: effects of an early structured psychiatric intervention, coping, and affective state on recurrence and survival 6 years later. Arch Gen Psychiatry 50:681–689, 1993

Frasure-Smith N, Lesperance F, Talajic M: Depression following myocardial infarction: impact on 6-month survival. JAMA 270:1819–1825, 1993

Guze SB, Daengsurisri S: Organic brain syndromes. Arch Gen Psychiatry 17:365–366, 1967

Hale M, Koss N, Kerstein M, et al: Psychiatric complications in a surgical ICU. Crit Care Med 5:199–203, 1977

Holmes TH, Rahe RH: The social readjustment rating scale. J Psychosom Res 11:213–218, 1967

Keitner GI, Ryan CE, Miller IW, et al: 12-month outcome of patients with major depression and comorbid psychiatric or medical illness (compound depression). Am J Psychiatry 148:345–350, 1991

Lazarus RS: Psychological Stress and the Coping Process. New York, McGraw-Hill, 1966

Linn L, Spitzer RL: DSM-III: implications for liaison psychiatry and psychosomatic medicine. JAMA 247:3207–3209, 1982

Lipowski ZJ: Psychosomatic medicine: past and present, I: historical background. Can J Psychiatry 31:2–7, 1986a

Lipowski ZJ: Psychosomatic medicine: past and present, III: current research. Can J Psychiatry 31:14–21, 1986b

Looney JG, Lipp MR, Spitzer RL: A new method of classification for psychophysiologic disorders. Am J Psychiatry 135:304–308, 1978

Meyer A: Psychobiology: A Science of Man. Springfield, IL, Charles C Thomas, 1957

Mezzich JE: International use and impact, in An Annotated Bibliography of DSM-III. Edited by Skodol AE, Spitzer RL. Washington, DC, American Psychiatric Press, 1987, pp 37–46

Morris PL, Raphael B, Robinson RG: Clinical depression is associated with impaired recovery from stroke. Med J Aust 157:239–242, 1992

Pavlov IP: The Work of the Digestive Glands. Translated by Thompson WH. Philadelphia, PA, JB Lippincott, 1902

Popkin MK: Disorders with physical symptoms, in An Annotated Bibliography of DSM-III. Edited by Skodol AE, Spitzer RL. Washington, DC, American Psychiatric Press, 1987, pp 74–75

Rosenman R, Brand R, Jenkins C, et al: Coronary heart disease in the Western Collaborative Group Study: final follow-up experience of eight and a half years. JAMA 233:872–877, 1975

Selye H: The general adaptation syndrome and the diseases of adaptation. J Clin Endocrinol 6:117–230, 1946

Silverstone PH: Depression increases mortality and morbidity in acute life-threatening medical illness. J Psychosom Res 34:651–657, 1990

Skodol AE: Problems in Differential Diagnosis: From DSM-III to DSM-III-R in Clinical Practice. Washington, DC, American Psychiatric Press, 1989

Spiegel DS, Kraemer HC, Bloom JR, et al: Effect of a psychosocial treatment on survival of patients with metastatic breast cancer. Lancet 2:888–891, 1989

Stoudemire A, Wallack L, Hedemark N: Alcohol dependence and abuse. American Journal of Preventive Medicine 3 (suppl 5):9–18, 1987a

Stoudemire A, Frank R, Kamlet M, et al: Depression. American Journal of Preventive Medicine 3 (suppl 5):65–71, 1987b

Stoudemire A, Strain JJ, Hales RE: DSM-IV issues for consultation psychiatry (editorial). Psychosomatics 30:239–244, 1989

Wells KB, Burnam MA: Caring for depression in America: lessons learned from early findings of the medical outcomes study. Psychiatr Med 9:503–519, 1991

Wells KB, Rogers W, Burnam MA, et al: Course of depression in patients with hypertension, myocardial infarction, or insulin-dependent diabetes. Am J Psychiatry 150:632–638 1993

Wolff HG: Stress and Disease. Springfield, IL, Charles C Thomas, 1953

CHAPTER 2

Cardiovascular Disease, Part I

Coronary Artery Disease
and Sudden Death

MICHAEL G. GOLDSTEIN, M.D.
RAYMOND NIAURA, PH.D.

Cardiovascular disease is considered in this chapter and in Chapter 3. In this chapter we cover the relationship of three psychological factors to coronary artery disease (CAD) and sudden death (including serious ventricular arrhythmias). These factors are personality or coping style, physiological hyperreactivity to environmental stimuli, and affective states. In Chapter 3 we complete the review of psychological factors affecting CAD and sudden death and then cover the area of hypertension. Subsections are devoted to discussions of the research linking specific psychological or behavioral factors with disease onset, exacerbation, or perpetuation. Evidence regarding the effectiveness of behavioral or psychosocial treatments is reviewed. Before describing the results of the literature review, we briefly describe some general theoretical issues that have characterized the research in this area. Theoretical issues specific to each psychological and behavioral factor are discussed in this chapter. The methods we have used for our literature review are also described. Finally, at the end of Chapter 3, we summarize the results of our review and provide recommendations for future research.

Theoretical Issues

In a comprehensive review of the literature, Dorian and Taylor (1984) developed a categorization of psychological factors affecting the development of CAD (Table 2–1). The psychological and behavioral factors that have been studied include affective states (e.g., anxiety, depression, acute situational disturbance), personality or coping style (e.g., Type A behavior pattern [TABP], components of TABP), physiological hyperreactivity to environmental stimuli (cardiovascular reactivity), sociocultural factors (e.g., work "overload," life stress), and interpersonal factors (e.g., lack of social support).

It must be noted that several of these factors are actually constructs made up of multiple components (e.g., TABP). Also, some factors have been defined by authors in varied ways, making collation and comparison of research findings somewhat difficult. Moreover, many of the research studies in this area have methodological deficiencies (e.g., nonrepresentative samples, failure to control for other variables that might affect outcome, measurement problems). Within the last several years, however, investigators have begun to address these problems. Recent research on the relationship between subcomponents of TABP and cardiovascular disease is an example of increased methodological sophistication (see subsection on TABP and subcomponents of TABP below).

TABLE 2–1.　Psychological and behavioral factors affecting coronary artery disease, sudden death, and ventricular arrhythmias

• **Affective states** 　Anxiety 　Depression 　Acute situational disturbance	• **Physiological hyperreactivity to environmental stimuli** 　Cardiovascular reactivity
• **Personality or coping style** 　Type A behavior pattern 　Components of Type A behavior 　　pattern 　　Hostility 　　"Anger-in"	• **Sociocultural factors** 　Work "overload" 　Other occupational factors 　Life stress • **Interpersonal factors** 　Lack of social support

Source.　Adapted from Dorian and Taylor 1984.

CAD and Sudden Death

In the following sections we review the literature that links psychological or behavioral factors with the development or outcome of CAD, sudden death, and serious ventricular arrhythmias.

Personality or Coping Style: TABP

Friedman (1969), a cardiologist, described and defined TABP in the 1960s after noting a high incidence of certain psychological traits and behaviors in clinical samples of patients with CAD. TABP is an "action-emotion complex," or a cluster of psychological and behavioral traits (see Table 2–2).

The relationship between TABP and CAD is complex. Krantz and Durel (1983) developed a model for understanding the relationship between TABP and CAD (Figure 2–1). As noted in Figure 2–1, the cognitive, behavioral, and emotional responses that characterize TABP are elicited by environmental challenges (Dorian and Taylor 1984). Furthermore, TABP contributes to the development of cardiovascular disease through its effect on physiological cardiovascular reactivity (Krantz and Durel 1983). Krantz and Durel also hypothesized that cognitive interpretation of physiological cardiovascular responses contributes to the expression of TABP. For example, an individual may interpret internal cues (e.g., palpitations, tremulousness) as signs of a threat and respond with increased TABP. Thus, the arrows between TABP and cardiovascular re-

---

TABLE 2–2.   Characteristics of the Type A behavior pattern

Hostility	Hard-driving behavior
Time urgency	Speech and motor characteristics
Impatience	Excessively rapid body movements
Aggressiveness	Tense facial and body musculature
Ambition	Explosive conversational speech
Competitiveness	Hand or teeth clenching
Setting excessively high performance	
standards	

Source.   Adapted from Friedman 1969.

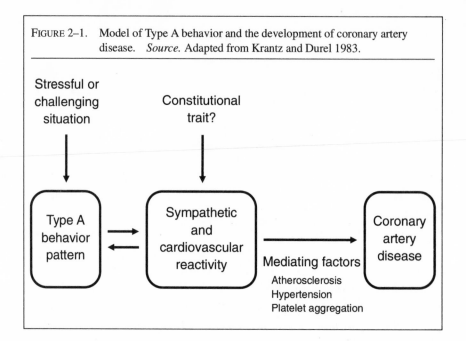

FIGURE 2–1. Model of Type A behavior and the development of coronary artery disease. *Source.* Adapted from Krantz and Durel 1983.

activity go both ways. Finally, genetic or constitutional factors may influence the expression of cardiovascular activity (Krantz and Durel 1983). Smith and Anderson (1986) added to this model by noting that individuals with TABP do not simply respond to environmental challenges and demands with typical cognitions, behaviors, and emotions; they also seek and create these challenging and stressful situations through their thoughts and behavior.

In a classic treatise, Price (1982) developed a comprehensive theoretical model, derived from social learning theory, to explain the development of TABP (Krantz and Durel 1983). To oversimplify greatly, Price posited that there are social, cultural, environmental, and personal antecedents to behavior (e.g., cultural beliefs, vehicles of socialization, physiological factors) that interact with cognitive and physiological factors to produce a core set of beliefs and fears (e.g., the belief that one must constantly prove oneself, the fear of insufficient supply). These, in turn lead to the development of overt manifestations of TABP. The social learning theory model also emphasizes that TABP is partially determined by the environmental and personal consequences of TABP that provide feedback to the individual and reinforce behavior (Price 1982).

TABP can be measured in several ways (Booth-Kewley and Friedman 1987). The Structured Interview (Rosenman 1978) uses a trained interviewer to ask questions pertinent to the definition in a deliberately challenging manner to bring out Type A behaviors. The Structured Interview measures both content and specific behaviors, including facial expressions, gestures, and speech characteristics. Although the Structured Interview has been used by most controlled studies that have used interviews to assess TABP, some studies have used a different script, with different indicators of Type A behavior and a different scoring procedure. The reader should bear this in mind when reviewing studies. Of the available self-report measures, the Jenkins Activity Survey (Jenkins et al. 1978) is best known. However, the Jenkins Activity Survey is relatively insensitive to behavioral components and underestimates the anger-hostility components of TABP (Krantz and Durel 1983).

Evidence documenting the presence of the relationships defined in Figure 2–1 are presented below. First, we review some of the evidence linking TABP with increased risk for developing CAD. Then, we present data on the relationship between *subcomponents* of TABP and CAD. Third, we present evidence linking TABP with increased sympathetic and cardiovascular physiological reactivity.

TABP: epidemiologic studies. Three major prospective studies have found TABP to be a risk factor for developing clinical CAD (French-Belgian Cooperative Group 1982; Haynes and Feinleib 1980; Rosenman et al. 1975). The Western Collaborative Group Study followed 3,200 employed men, all without a history of CAD at the start of the study, for 8.5 years (Rosenman et al. 1975). The study found that Type A men had twice the incidence of CAD as Type B men. This association held even after the effects of traditional risk factors were controlled statistically. Results from the Framingham Heart Study indicated that Type A behavior is an independent predictor of the 8-year incidence of CAD and myocardial infarction (MI) among men, but only among those with white-collar positions (Haynes and Feinleib 1980). TABP was also predictive of CAD in women 45–64 years of age (Haynes and Feinleib 1980). The French-Belgian Cooperative Group study also found TABP to be an independent predictor of total CAD, MI, and sudden death. The French-Belgian Cooperative study was based on a 5-year study of initially healthy men from

European communities. However, the positive results of these three studies are tempered by a more recent analysis of the data from the Western Collaborative Group Study, which revealed that global TABP was not a significant predictor of CAD mortality after either 8.5 or 22 years of follow-up (Ragland and Brand 1988).

The three studies described above all involved initially healthy individuals without CAD. Three longitudinal studies of patients with either a previous MI or elevated traditional risk factors found no association between TABP measures and subsequent CAD (Case et al. 1985; Shekelle et al. 1985a, 1985b). Moreover, Rosenman (1985) reported that Type A subjects in the Western Collaborative Group Study who had an MI actually had less subsequent mortality at follow-up than Type B subjects. The results of these studies are reflected in the report of a meta-analysis of the association of TABP and CAD published in 1988 (Matthews 1988); Matthews found that the association of global TABP and CAD was significant only in those studies that had a population-based sample. There was not a significant association between TABP and CAD events in studies of patients at high risk for CAD (Matthews 1988). More recent studies have also supported this finding (Ahern et al. 1990; Barefoot et al. 1989b). However, another study of recurrent cardiac events found that although TABP was not a significant predictor of nonsudden cardiac death or nonfatal recurrent events, it was a significant predictor of sudden cardiac death (Brackett and Powell 1988).

To summarize, epidemiologic evidence suggests that TABP is a risk factor for the *development* of CAD, but recent evidence suggests that once CAD is present or risk is high, the presence of global TABP does not increase the risk of having subsequent morbid events, except perhaps sudden cardiac death. These findings have led to a search for components of TABP that may be more strongly associated with CAD.

TABP: angiography studies.   A number of studies have demonstrated a relationship between TABP and the extent of coronary atherosclerosis as measured by coronary angiogram (Blumenthal et al. 1978; Frank et al. 1978; Williams et al. 1988; Zyzanski et al. 1976). However, in a 1985 review of the literature, Pickering found no consistent relationship between *overall* TABP and extent of CAD as measured by coronary angiography. In a study of more than 2,200 patients, Williams and colleagues

(1988) found that TABP, when measured by the Structured Interview, was significantly associated with CAD severity after other risk factors were controlled for. However, this relationship was present only in patients age 45 years or younger.

Pickering (1985) described a number of confounding factors present in studies of this type, which may explain the discrepancies found. Among these are differences in methods, bias in the selection of subjects, and the lack of a true control group. As Pickering also pointed out, the only coronary risk factor that has been consistently associated with extent of atherosclerosis, as measured by angiogram, is hypercholesterolemia. He concluded that measuring atherosclerosis by coronary angiogram should not be the "gold standard" for assessing the role of behavioral factors in the development of CAD. Miller and colleagues (1988) suggested methods to deal with the biases inherent in studying referred samples, such as patients presenting for angiographic study. In a 1991 commentary, Pearson and Derby suggested that such studies still have a role in defining associations between risk factors and CAD. Subsequent studies that have explored the relationship between components of TABP and angiographically defined CAD have reported positive relationships (Dembroski et al. 1985; Siegman et al. 1987).

TABP: components of Type A.   Over the last decade, investigators have moved away from measuring global TABP and have attempted to identify the components of TABP that are most strongly associated with CAD. Here we review briefly the evidence from the studies resulting from this effort. For a more complete discussion of this topic, readers are referred elsewhere (Dembroski et al. 1989; Manuck et al. 1986; Williams and Anderson 1987).

The Cook-Medley Hostility Inventory (Cook and Medley 1954), which is derived from the Minnesota Multiphasic Personality Inventory (MMPI) (Hathaway and McKinley 1943), is a psychometric measure of hostility that has been found to be predictive of CAD events and total mortality in three prospective studies (Barefoot et al. 1983, 1989a; Shekelle et al. 1983). The association was independent of the traditional risk factors. In the Western Electric study, 1,877 middle-aged men completed the MMPI at baseline and were followed for coronary heart disease (CHD) events over a 10-year period (Shekelle et al. 1983). Results showed that CHD event rate increased as a function of higher hostility scores in this population. In another study, Barefoot and colleagues (1983) followed 255 physicians for a 25-year period. Physicians completed the MMPI at baseline. Results showed that higher hostility scores at baseline were associated with an almost fivefold higher risk of CHD events during the follow-up period. In a third prospective study, Barefoot and colleagues (1989a) followed 118 law students for 25 years. Hostility scores at baseline were related to risk of all-cause mortality in a linear fashion, with higher scores predicting greater risk. This study also suggests that subsets of items from the Cook-Medley scale, representing cynicism, hostile affect, and aggressive response, were more strongly related to survival than was the full-scale score.

Almada and colleagues (1991) found that an MMPI-derived cynicism scale, closely related to the cynicism component of the Cook-Medley scale, predicted coronary death and total mortality in a subset of men participating in the Western Electric study. They also found that increased hostility was related to increased cigarette smoking and alcohol consumption. Other studies have also noted that Cook-Medley hostility scores are related to poor health habits, including less physical activity, smoking, drinking alcohol, greater body mass index, greater caloric intake, and increased caffeine consumption (Smith 1992). These studies collectively suggest that risk of CAD and mortality due to cynical hostility may be attributable in part to the effects of excessive unhealthy behaviors.

The results of these prospective investigations must be viewed with caution, however, because three studies have failed to replicate these findings (Hearn et al. 1989; Leon et al. 1988; McCranie et al. 1986). However, methodological differences among the studies may explain some of the discrepant results (Dembroski et al. 1989). The Cook-Medley Hostility Scale, the measure of hostility used in the studies described above, is thought to assess suspiciousness, resentment, frequent anger, and cynical mistrust of others, rather than overtly aggressive behavior or general emotional distress (Smith and Frohm 1985). Individuals who score high on this index of hostility are less hardy, display more anger, experience more frequent and severe hassles, and have fewer and less satisfactory social supports. Barefoot and colleagues (1989a) analyzed the construct validity of the hostility scale and derived a subset of items that included having a cynical attitude toward others, frequently experiencing anger, and responding to frustration with aggression.

"Potential for hostility," a behavioral rating derived from the Structured Interview, has been implicated as specifically pathogenic for CAD and CHD (Dembroski et al. 1989). Potential for hostility reflects hostile content of answers, intensity of hostile responses, and hostile style of interaction with the interviewer (Dembroski and MacDougall 1983). The results of two angiographic studies have supported a relationship between potential for hostility and extent of CAD, independent of other risk factors. A study of 131 patients drawn randomly from more than 2,000 patients undergoing coronary angiography found that both potential for hostility and "anger-in," a behaviorally rated measure of anger inhibition derived from the Structured Interview, predicted disease severity (Dembroski et al. 1985). Of interest was the finding that potential for hostility was related to CAD outcome measures only when high anger-in was also present, thus suggesting that the combination of high hostility and inhibition of anger expression was pathogenic for CAD. Another study by the same group of investigators on another angiographic sample replicated their finding of significant correlations between potential for hostility and severity of CAD (MacDougall et al. 1985). In contrast to the previous study, however, potential for hostility and anger-in did not interact in predicting extent of CAD.

Several prospective investigations also indicated that measures of hostility and anger are also related to incidence of CHD (Smith 1992). Matthews and colleagues (1977) found that behaviorally based Structured Interview ratings of potential for hostility were prospectively associated with CHD in the Western Collaborative Group Study. Hecker and colleagues (1988) also compared CHD cases and matched controls on TABP components in the Western Collaborative Group Study after an 8.5-year follow-up period. They found that, of all component ratings derived from the Structured Interview, potential for hostility was the best predictor of CHD incidence, independent of other traditional risk factors. In the Framingham sample, anger-in (not expressing anger outwardly) predicted an 8-year incidence of CAD among women and white-collar men (Manuck et al. 1986). In a study of 3,750 Finnish men 39–59 years of age, high ratings of hostility (assessed from self-ratings of irritability, ease of anger-arousal, and argumentativeness) significantly increased the risk of total mortality, mainly due to ischemic heart disease during a 3-year follow-up (Koskenvuo et al. 1988). However, the relationship between hostility and mortality was confined to men with preexisting hypertension or ischemic heart disease. This last study suggests that hostility may combine with preexisting physiological cardiac risk factors to increase mortality risk.

Some studies have suggested that there may be particular aspects of hostility that are more pathogenic than the overall construct. Siegman and colleagues (1987) performed a factor analysis of the Buss-Durkee Hostility Inventory (Buss and Durkee 1957) and identified two factors: neurotic hostility and expressive hostility. These measures were administered to a sample of patients undergoing coronary angiography. The results show that neurotic hostility was significantly but inversely related to CAD severity, whereas expressive hostility was significantly and positively related to CAD severity. Thus, it appears that expressive aspects of hostility are especially pathogenic for CAD. Dembroski and colleagues (1989) tested the hypothesis that hostility is associated with increased relative risk for coronary death and nonfatal MI among participants in the Multiple Risk Factor Intervention Trial. After a 7-year follow-up period, 192 CAD patients were compared with 384 matched, nondiseased control subjects on a variety of characteristics associated with a TABP, including three different but interrelated components of hostility. Total ratings of potential for hostility were related to incidence of CHD. However, a rating of "stylistic hostility," a subcomponent of potential for hostility, showed the most significant association with CHD incidence, independent of traditional risk factors. The stylistic hostility subcomponent reflects an antagonistic interactional style noted during the Structured Interview assessment for TABP (Dembroski et al. 1989).

To summarize, expressive hostility, and antagonistic interactions in particular, appear to be the subcomponents of TABP that are most strongly related to risk of CAD and CHD. Other measures of hostility also have been found to predict CAD morbidity and mortality, including cynical mistrust of others and the affective experience of anger. The effects of hostility on coronary disease may be mediated by its effects on other risk behaviors, such as smoking or alcohol consumption (Smith 1992). Increased hostility is also associated with certain demographic characteristics, such as nonwhite race, low socioeconomic status, male gender, and low level of education (Barefoot et al. 1991; Scherwitz et al. 1991). Because this distribution of hostility scores closely mirrors the pattern of health in the population, hostility may be one of the risk factors that explain the uneven distribution of disease in the population (Barefoot et al. 1991; Scherwitz et al. 1991).

Treatment of TABP and CAD outcome.   In a meta-analysis of 18 controlled studies of the effect of psychological treatment of TABP, Nunes and colleagues (1987) found that psychological treatment aimed at reducing TABP led to a reduction in TABP measures by about half a standard deviation, which the authors considered to be a moderately large effect size compared with the treatment intervention literature as a whole. These investigators also performed a meta-analysis of the effect of psychological treatment of TABP on clinical outcome of coronary heart disease and found that there was a marginally significant effect of treatment on the combination of coronary events and mortality at 1 year. However, they also found that the two studies that obtained 3-year follow-up data reported a 50% reduction in coronary events, a highly significant effect.

The investigators from the Recurrent Coronary Prevention Project, one of the two long-term studies reviewed in the meta-analysis, published 4.5-year follow-up results (Powell and Thoresen 1988). After 3 years, the addition of Type A counseling to standard counseling for post-MI patients had resulted in significant reductions in Type A behavior and a 44% lower rate of recurrence (nonfatal MI and coronary death) (Friedman et al. 1984). After 4.5 years, the relationship between Type A counseling and reduced nonfatal MI was maintained, but only those subjects with good functional status were protected from cardiac death by Type A counseling (Powell and Thoresen 1988). Type A counseling resulted in significant reductions in Type A components, such as hostility, time urgency, and impatience, and it also significantly decreased depression and anger and increased social support and well-being (Mendes de Leon et al. 1991). These results suggest that Type A counseling's specific and nonspecific beneficial effects were mediators of its efficacy. Although the number of studies remains small, it appears that psychological treatment of TABP improves clinical outcome.

Physiological Hyperreactivity to Environmental Stimuli: Psychophysiological Correlates of TABP

As noted earlier, it has been hypothesized that TABP contributes to the development of CAD through its effect on sympathetic and cardiovascular reactivity (see Figure 2–1). TABP is believed to lead to repeated and excessive activation of potentially pathogenic neuroendocrine and cardiovascular responses (Krantz and Durel 1983; Manuck et al. 1986). There are numerous studies that report that TABP subjects frequently display larger episodic increases in blood pressure, heart rate, and catecholamines when confronted by challenging or stressful tasks (Krantz and Durel 1983; Manuck et al. 1986; Williams et al. 1991). Although the challenging nature of the task is felt to be an important mediating factor in demonstrating greater reactivity in TABP, these subjects also have been noted to have greater systolic blood pressure reactivity when unconscious during coronary bypass surgery (Krantz and Durel 1983). Components of TABP, such as hostility, are also associated with greater cardiovascular reactivity (Dembroski et al. 1979; Glass et al. 1983; Smith and Allred 1989; Suarez and Williams 1989; Weidner et al. 1989). A discussion of the relationships between cardiovascular reactivity, TABP, and hypertension is provided in Chapter 3.

There is now considerable evidence that activation of the sympathetic nervous system during behavioral challenge contributes to the development of atherosclerosis and clinical coronary disease (Krantz and Manuck 1984; Manuck et al. 1986, 1989; Niaura et al. 1992). The best evidence for this comes from primate studies. Manuck and colleagues (1986, 1989) reported that monkeys with high reactivity to a standard stressor (threat of capture) develop twice the extent of coronary atherosclerosis as low-reactive animals when fed a moderately atherogenic diet. Both hemodynamic mechanisms (e.g., hypertension, increased turbulence) and neuroendocrine mechanisms (e.g., catecholaminergic influences on platelet aggregation and vascular tone) have been hypothesized to mediate the relationship between cardiovascular reactivity and CAD, but the mechanisms have not been fully elucidated (Barefoot et al. 1983; Manuck et al. 1986; Markovitz and Matthews 1991). Also, it should be noted that studies with humans attempting to link physiological reactivity to stress and CAD are few and inconsistent (Keys et al. 1971; Manuck et al. 1992; Russek et al. 1990). However, the evidence that links TABP and components of TABP to cardiovascular reactivity provides further indirect evidence linking these constructs to the development of cardiovascular disease.

Affective States

Depression. Patients with an untreated major depressive episode have an increased risk for cardiovascular mortality, especially from sudden death (Avery and Winokur 1976; Murphy et al. 1987). Carney and colleagues (1988b) demonstrated that a DSM-III (American Psychiatric Association 1980) diagnosis of major depressive disorder, derived from the Diagnostic Interview Schedule, is the best predictor of major cardiac events (e.g., myocardial infarction, angioplasty, coronary artery bypass surgery, death) during the 12 months after cardiac catheterization. This effect was independent of the severity of CAD, left ventricular ejection fraction, and smoking. Other studies have noted that major depressive disorder in both cardiac and noncardiac patients is associated with increased sympathetic nervous system activity (Carney et al. 1988a; Esler et al. 1982), suggesting a possible mechanism for increased risk of coronary events in patients with preexisting cardiac disease.

Therefore, there is good evidence that patients with a major depressive disorder are at increased risk for a cardiovascular morbidity and mortality. Clearly, one cannot generalize from these results and assume that individuals with depressive symptoms that do not meet the criteria for major depressive disorder would also have greater risk of cardiovascular morbidity. However, the results of three studies that have focused on the relationship between depressive symptoms and cardiac disease demonstrated that self-reported depressive symptoms are correlated with sudden death (Bruhn et al. 1974), severe ventricular arrhythmias (Orth-Gomér et al. 1980), and cardiac arrest (Ahern et al. 1990).

Other studies have looked at the relationship between patients' depressive symptoms or mood and CAD outcomes. Booth-Kewley and Friedman (1987) performed a meta-analysis of this literature (13 studies) and concluded that depression is related to CHD outcomes (i.e., global MI, angina, cardiac death) with an effect size that is higher than that for TABP (Booth-Kewley and Friedman 1987). When an analysis was performed separately for the six prospective studies, depression again was strongly related to CAD outcome, suggesting a causal link (Booth-Kewley and Friedman 1987). However, a more recent meta-analysis by Matthews (1988), which was more conservative in selecting studies for analysis and which weighted studies according to the number of participants, found that depression was not a predictor of CAD.

Thus, although there is clearly an association between the presence of a clinical depressive disorder and cardiovascular morbidity and mortality, the relationship between patients' depressive symptoms and cardiovascular disease outcomes is less clear. The best evidence for such a relationship can be found for such outcomes as severe ventricular arrhythmias, cardiac arrest, and sudden death; more research is needed to establish a relationship between depressive symptoms and other cardiovascular disease endpoints.

Anxiety.   Booth-Kewley and Friedman (1987) also performed a meta-analysis of studies of the relationship between patient anxiety and CHD outcomes. They included 15 studies in their meta-analysis and concluded that anxiety is only slightly related to CHD outcomes. Moreover, only 3 of the 15 studies were prospective. When Booth-Kewley and Friedman performed a separate meta-analysis of the studies published after 1977, they found no significant relationship between patient anxiety and outcomes. Matthews (1988), using conservative criteria in selecting studies for her meta-analysis, could find only two studies of anxiety that met her criteria, and only one of these reported significant positive relationships. The outcome measure for this study was angina, a soft outcome measure because it is based on patient reports of chest pain (Matthews 1988). Thus, we conclude that the relationship between anxiety symptoms and other measures of patient anxiety and the development and progression of CAD is unclear.

In Chapter 3 we continue our discussion of psychological factors affecting CAD and sudden death by focusing on acute situational disturbances. It appears that acute distress occurring in the setting of a disturbing life event is an important factor in triggering serious ventricular arrhythmias and sudden death in patients who are predisposed to these cardiac events. Anxiety associated with an acute MI and cardiac surgery is also briefly discussed in Chapter 3.

References

Ahern DK, Gorkin L, Anderson JL, et al: Biobehavioral variables and mortality or cardiac arrest in the Cardiac Arrhythmia Pilot Study (CAPS). Am J Cardiol 66:59–62, 1990

Almada SJ, Zonderman AB, Shekelle RB, et al: Neuroticism and cynicism and risk of death in middle-aged men: the Western Electric Study. Psychosom Med 53:165–175, 1991

American Psychiatric Association: Diagnostic and Statistical Manual of Mental Disorders, 3rd Edition. Washington, DC, American Psychiatric Association, 1980

Avery D, Winokur G: Mortality in depressed patients treated with electroconvulsive therapy and antidepressants. Arch Gen Psychiatry 33:1029–1037, 1976

Barefoot JC, Dahlstrom WC, Williams RB: Hostility, CHD incidence and total mortality: a 25-year follow-up study of 255 physicians. Psychosom Med 45:59–63, 1983

Barefoot JC, Dodge KA, Peterson BL, et al: The Cook-Medley Hostility Scale: item content and ability to predict survival. Psychosom Med 51:46–57, 1989a

Barefoot JC, Peterson BC, Harrell FE Jr, et al: Type A behavior and survival: a follow-up study of 1,467 patients with coronary artery disease. Am J Cardiol 64:427–432, 1989b

Barefoot JC, Peterson BL, Dahlstrom WG, et al: Hostility patterns and health implications: correlates of Cook-Medley Hostility Scale scores in a national survey. Health Psychol 10:18–24, 1991

Blumenthal JA, Williams RB, Kong Y, et al: Type A behavior pattern and coronary atherosclerosis. Circulation 58:634–639, 1978

Booth-Kewley S, Friedman HS: Psychological predictors of heart disease: a quantitative review. Psychol Bull 101:343–362, 1987

Brackett CD, Powell LH: Psychosocial and physiological predictors of sudden cardiac death after healing of acute myocardial infarction. Am J Cardiol 61:979–983, 1988

Bruhn J, Paredes A, Adsert C, et al: Psychosocial predictors of sudden death in myocardial infarction. J Psychosom Res 18:187–191, 1974

Buss AH, Durkee A: An inventory of assessing different kinds of hostility. Journal of Consulting Psychology 21:343–349, 1957

Carney RM, Rich MW, teVelde A, et al: Heart rate, heart rate variability and depression in patients with coronary artery disease. J Psychosom Res 32:159–164, 1988a

Carney RM, Rich MW, Freedland KE, et al: Major depressive disorder predicts cardiac events in patients with coronary artery disease. Psychosom Med 50:627–633, 1988b

Case RB, Heller SS, Case NB, et al: Type A behavior and survival after acute myocardial infarction. N Engl J Med 312:737–741, 1985

Cook W, Medley D: Proposed hostility and pharisaic-virtue scales for the MMPI. J Appl Psychol 238:414–418, 1954

Dembroski TM, MacDougall JM: Behavioral and psychophysiological perspectives on coronary-prone behavior, in Biobehavioral Bases of Coronary Heart Disease. Edited by Dembroski TM, Schmidt TN, Blumchen G. New York, Karger, 1983, pp 106–129

Dembroski TM, MacDougall JM, Herd JA, et al: Effects of level of challenge on pressor and heart rate responses in Type A and Type B subjects. Journal of Applied Social Psychology 9:208–228, 1979

Dembroski TM, MacDougall JM, Williams RB, et al: Components of Type A, hostility, and anger-in: relationship to angiographic findings. Psychosom Med 47:219–233, 1985

Dembroski TM, MacDougall JM, Costa PT, et al: Components of hostility as predictors of sudden death and myocardial infarction in the Multiple Risk Factor Intervention Trial. Psychosom Med 51:514–522, 1989

Dorian B, Taylor CB: Stress factors in the development of coronary artery disease. J Occup Med 26:747–756, 1984

Esler M, Turbott J, Schwartz R, et al: The peripheral kinetics of norepinephrine in depressive illness. Arch Gen Psychiatry 39:285–300, 1982

Frank KA, Heller SS, Kornfeld DS, et al: Type A behavior pattern and coronary angiographic findings. JAMA 240:761–763, 1978

French-Belgian Cooperative Group: Ischemic heart disease and psychological patterns: prevalence and incidence studies in Belgium and France. Adv Cardiol 29:25–31, 1982

Friedman M: Pathogenesis of Coronary Artery Disease. New York, McGraw-Hill, 1969

Friedman M, Thoresen CE, Gill JJ, et al: Alteration of Type A behavior and reduction in cardiac recurrences in postmyocardial infarction patients. Am Heart J 108:237–248, 1984

Glass DC, Lake CR, Contrada RJ, et al: Stability of individual differences in physiological responses to stress. Health Psychol 2:317–341, 1983

Hathaway SR, McKinley JC: Minnesota Multiphasic Personality Inventory. Minneapolis, MN, University of Minnesota, 1943

Haynes SG, Feinleib M: Women, work, and coronary heart disease: prospective findings from the Framingham heart study. Am J Public Health 70:133–141, 1980

Hearn MD, Murray DM, Luepker RV: Hostility, coronary heart disease and total mortality: a 33-year follow-up study of university students. J Behav Med 12:105–121, 1989

Hecker MHL, Chesney MA, Black GW, et al: Coronary-prone behaviors in the Western Collaborative Group Study. Psychosom Med 50:153–164, 1988

Jenkins CD, Zyzanski SK, Rosenman RH: Coronary-prone behavior: one pattern or several? Psychosom Med 40:24–43, 1978

Keys A, Taylor HL, Blackburn H, et al: Mortality and coronary heart disease among men studied for 23 years. Arch Intern Med 128:201–214, 1971

Koskenvuo M, Kaprio J, Rose RJ, et al: Hostility as a risk factor for mortality and ischemic heart disease in men. Psychosom Med 50:330–340, 1988

Krantz DS, Durel LA: Psychobiological substrates of the Type A behavior pattern. Health Psychol 2:393–411, 1983

Krantz DS, Manuck SB: Acute psychophysiologic reactivity and risk of cardiovascular disease: a review and methodologic critique. Psychol Bull 96:435–464, 1984

Leon GR, Finn SE, Murray D, et al: Inability to predict cardiovascular disease from hostility scores or MMPI items related to Type A behavior. J Consult Clin Psychol 56:597–600, 1988

MacDougall JM, Dembroski TM, Dimsdale JE, et al: Components of Type A, hostility, and anger-in: further relationships to angiographic findings. Health Psychol 4:137–152, 1985

Manuck SB, Kaplan JR, Matthews KA: Behavioral antecedents of coronary heart disease and atherosclerosis. Arteriosclerosis 6:2–14, 1986

Manuck SB, Kaplan JR, Adams MR, et al: Behaviorally elicited heart rate reactivity and atherosclerosis in female Cynomologus monkeys (*Macaca fascicularis*). Psychosom Med 51:306–318, 1989

Manuck SB, Olsson G, Hjemdahl P, et al: Does cardiovascular reactivity to mental stress have prognostic value in postinfarction patients? a pilot study. Psychosom Med 55:37–43, 1992

Markovitz JH, Matthews KA: Platelets and coronary heart disease: potential psychophysiologic mechanisms. Psychosom Med 53:643–668, 1991

Matthews KA: Coronary heart disease and Type A behaviors: update on and alternative to the Booth-Kewley and Friedman (1987) quantitative review. Psychol Bull 104:373–380, 1988

Matthews KA, Glass DC, Rosenman RH, et al: Competitive drive, pattern A, and coronary heart disease: a further analysis of some data from the Western Collaborative Group Study. Journal of Chronic Disease 30:489–498, 1977

McCranie EW, Watkins L, Brandsma J, et al: Hostility, coronary heart disease (CHD) incidence, and total mortality: lack of association in a 25-year follow-up study of 478 physicians. J Behav Med 9:119–125, 1986

Mendes de Leon CF, Powell LH, Kaplan BH: Change in coronary-prone behaviors in the Recurrent Coronary Preventions Project. Psychosom Med 53:407–419, 1991

Miller TQ, Turner CW, Tindale RS, et al: Disease based spectrum bias in referred samples and the relationship between Type A behavior and coronary artery disease. J Clin Epidemiol 41:1139–1149, 1988

Murphy JM, Monson PR, Olivier DC, et al: Affective disorders and mortality: a general population study. Arch Gen Psychiatry 44:473–480, 1987

Niaura R, Stoney CM, Herbert PN: Lipids in psychological research: the last decade. Biol Psychol 34:1–43, 1992

Nunes EV, Frank KA, Kornfeld DS: Psychologic treatment for the Type A behavior pattern and for coronary heart disease: a meta analysis of the literature. Psychosom Med 48:159–173, 1987

Orth-Gomér K, Edwards ME, Erhardt L, et al: Relation between ventricular arrhythmias and psychologic profile. Acta Medica Scandinavica 207:31–36, 1980

Pearson TA, Derby CA: Invited commentary: should arteriographic case-control studies be used to identify causes of atherosclerotic coronary artery disease? Am J Epidemiol 134:123–128, 1991

Pickering TG: Should studies of patients undergoing coronary angiography be used to evaluate the role of behavioral risk factors for coronary heart disease? J Behav Med 8:203–213, 1985

Powell LH, Thoresen CE: Effects of Type A behavioral counseling and severity of prior acute myocardial infarction on survival. Am J Cardiol 62:1159–1163, 1988

Price VA: Type A Behavior Pattern: A Model for Research and Practice. New York, Academic Press, 1982

Ragland DR, Brand RJ: Type A behavior and mortality from coronary heart disease. N Engl J Med 318:65–69, 1988

Rosenman RH: The interview method of assessment of the coronary-prone behavior pattern, in Coronary-Prone Behavior. Edited by Dembroski TM, Weiss S, Shields J, et al. New York, Springer-Verlag, 1978, pp 55–69

Rosenman RH: The impact of anxiety on the cardiovascular system. Psychosomatics 26 (suppl):6–15, 1985

Rosenman RH, Brand RJ, Jenkins CD, et al: Coronary heart disease in the Western Collaborative Group Study: final follow-up experience of eight and one-half years. JAMA 233:872–877, 1975

Russek LG, King SH, Russek SJ, et al: The Harvard Mastery of Stress Study 35-year follow-up: prognostic significance of patterns of psychophysiological arousal and adaption. Psychosom Med 52:271–285, 1990

Scherwitz L, Perkins L, Chesney M, et al: Cook-Medley Hostility Scale and subsets: relationship to demographic and psychosocial characteristics in young adults in the CARDIA study. Psychosom Med 53:36–49, 1991

Shekelle RB, Gale M, Ostfield A, et al: Hostility, risk of coronary heart disease, and mortality. Psychosom Med 45:109–114, 1983

Shekelle RB, Gale M, Norusis M: For the Aspirin Myocardial Infarction Study Research Group: Type A score (Jenkins Activity Survey) and risk of recurrent coronary heart disease in the Aspirin Myocardial Infarction Study. Am J Cardiol 56:221–225, 1985a

Shekelle RB, Hulley SB, Neaton J, et al: The MRFIT behavioral pattern study, I: Type A behavior pattern and risk of coronary death in MRFIT. Am J Epidemiol 122:559–570, 1985b

Siegman AW, Dembroski TM, Ringel N: Components of hostility and the severity of coronary artery disease. Psychosom Med 49:127–135, 1987

Smith TW: Hostility and health: current status of a psychosomatic hypothesis. Health Psychol 11:139–150, 1992

Smith TW, Allred KD: Blood-pressure responses during social interaction in high- and low-cynically hostile males. J Behav Med 12:135–143, 1989

Smith TW, Anderson NB: Models of personality and disease: an interactional approach to Type A behavior and cardiovascular risk. J Pers Soc Psychol 50:1166–1173, 1986

Smith TW, Frohm KD: What's so unhealthy about hostility? construct validity and psychosocial correlates of the Cook and Medley Ho Scale. Health Psychol 4:503–520, 1985

Suarez EC, Williams RB Jr: Situational determinants of cardiovascular and emotional reactivity in high and low hostile men. Psychosom Med 51:404–418, 1989

Weidner G, Friend R, Ficarrotto TJ, et al: Hostility and cardiovascular reactivity to stress in women and men. Psychosom Med 51:36–45, 1989

Williams RB, Anderson NB: Hostility and coronary heart disease, in Cardiovascular Disease and Behavior. Edited by Elias JW, Marshall PH. Washington, DC, Hemisphere/Harper & Row, 1987, pp 17–37

Williams RB, Barefoot JC, Haney TL, et al: Type A behavior and angiographically documented coronary atherosclerosis in a sample of 2,289 patients. Psychosom Med 50:139–152, 1988

Williams R Jr, Suarez EC, Kuhn CM, et al: Biobehavioral basis of coronary-prone behavior in middle-aged men, part I: evidence for chronic SNS activation in Type As. Psychosom Med 53:517–527, 1991

Zyzanski SJ, Jenkins CD, Ryan TJ, et al: Psychological correlates of coronary angiographic findings. Arch Intern Med 136:1234–1237, 1976

CHAPTER 3

Cardiovascular Disease, Part II

Coronary Artery Disease and Sudden Death and Hypertension

RAYMOND NIAURA, PH.D.
MICHAEL G. GOLDSTEIN, M.D.

In this chapter we continue the discussion of the relationship between psychological factors affecting coronary artery disease (CAD) and sudden death. The results of research on the relationship between acute situational disturbances—defined here as acutely disturbing stressful life events or situations—and cardiovascular disease outcomes are discussed. The literature on ventricular arrhythmias and sudden death as well as work regarding the relationship between mental stress and myocardial ischemia are reviewed. We consider acute situational disturbances by briefly discussing the stress associated with being a patient in an intensive care or coronary care unit, and we conclude with a discussion of sociocultural and interpersonal factors.

Acute Situational Disturbance

Sudden Death and Ventricular Arrhythmias

A number of studies have demonstrated a connection between sudden death and acute disturbing life events (Dorian and Taylor 1984; Fricchione and Vlay 1986; Greene et al. 1972; Kamarck and Jennings 1991; Myers and Dewar 1975; Reich et al. 1981; Siltanen 1978; Tavazzi et al.

1986). For example, Reich and colleagues found that the onset of malignant ventricular arrhythmias was associated with identifiable emotional triggers in 21% of patients referred for antiarrhythmic management. In a group of patients with the long QT syndrome, a condition that increases vulnerability to serious cardiac arrhythmias, Schwartz (1984) clearly documented the arrhythmogenic effects of stress-induced sympathetic arousal. Follick and colleagues (1988) demonstrated that distress during hospitalization for a myocardial infarction (MI) predicted the presence of ventricular arrhythmias on ambulatory electrocardiograms obtained during the year following the infarction.

Several studies have shown that psychological stress, induced in an experimental paradigm, will increase the number of ventricular premature beats in patients with preexisting ventricular arrhythmias as well as lower thresholds for ventricular fibrillation (Lown and DeSilva 1978; Tavazzi et al. 1986). However, except for the study by Follick and colleagues (1988) mentioned above, there are no controlled prospective studies in clinically relevant populations documenting the relationship between psychological precipitants and significant ventricular arrhythmias or sudden death. Moreover, a more recent report by Follick and colleagues (1990) describing another sample of post-MI patients reported no significant relationship between psychological measures and ventricular arrhythmias assessed at 3, 6, and 13 months after enrollment.

Lown (1987) developed a model for the development of life-threatening ventricular fibrillation that depicts the interaction of three factors: 1) ventricular electrical instability, which is increased in the presence of ischemic heart disease; 2) psychological state (e.g., depression, Type A behavior pattern [TABP]); and 3) triggers (e.g., emotional events, public speaking, automobile driving, and other acute stresses). In a comprehensive review of biobehavioral factors in sudden cardiac death, Kamarck and Jennings (1991) proposed an expanded model for understanding the psychophysiology of sudden death (Figure 3–1). Their model links psychological factors with activation of the autonomic nervous system, which in turn produces physiological changes that promote the development of cardiac arrhythmias. According to this model, psychological factors and resulting autonomic activation influence the development of sudden death at three levels: 1) through the promotion of CAD (e.g., atherosclerosis), 2) by influencing "priming processes" (i.e., coronary vasospasm, platelet aggregation, and plaque rupture), and 3) by directly triggering lethal arrhythmias (i.e., ventricular tachyarrhythmias and bradyrhythmias). Schwartz and colleagues (1992) provided evidence that vagal activity may have a protective effect on ventricular arrhythmias. The model proposed by Kamarck and Jennings can help to guide recommendations for further research in this area. These authors have identified five areas for future research initiatives: 1) epidemiologic field research to investigate the relationship between life stressors and sudden cardiac death, 2) clinical research focusing on the relationship between acute psychological stressors and ambulatory arrhythmias and ischemia, 3) laboratory research that focuses on the patterns of autonomic activity (e.g., neurohumoral, hemodynamic) associated with response to acute stressors, 4) research attempting to identify the relationship between individual differences in autonomic tone or cardiovascular reactivity and vulnerability to sudden cardiac death, and 5) examination of the effects of psychological or behaviorally based treatment in patients at high risk for sudden cardiac death (Kamarck and Jennings 1991). Dimsdale and colleagues (1987) identified a similar research agenda for this area.

FIGURE 3–1. Pathways of psychological influences in sudden cardiac death. *Source.* Adapted from Kamarck and Jennings 1991.

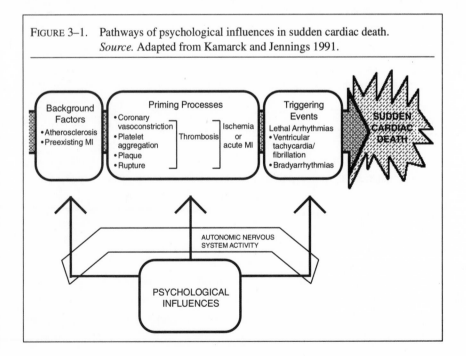

Mental Stress and Myocardial Ischemia

Myocardial ischemia develops when myocardial demands for oxygen increase to a level exceeding the capacity of diseased coronary arteries to deliver blood or when coronary vasoconstriction increases so that flow decreases to critical levels (Epstein et al. 1988). The relationship between symptoms of myocardial ischemia, angina pectoris, and mental stress has been well recognized (Deanfield et al. 1984). It has been demonstrated that asymptomatic, or "silent," myocardial ischemia is relatively common in patients with CAD and may be precipitated by both physical stress and mental stress (Deanfield et al. 1984; Rozanski et al. 1988; Selwyn and Ganz 1988). In an experimental study, Rozanski and colleagues studied the comparative effects of different forms of mental stress in 39 patients with CAD and found that 59% had evidence of ischemia during periods of mental stress (i.e., mental arithmetic, the Stroop color-word test, simulated public speaking) and that ischemia induced by mental stress was silent in 83% of these episodes. Moreover, the magnitude of the abnormalities noted during the most potent mental stress (public speaking) was not significantly different from that induced by vigorous exercise in the same patients (Rozanski et al. 1988). Other studies using new and sensitive cardiac imaging techniques, such as echocardiography and radionuclide detectors, have also demonstrated the effects of mental stress on cardiac function (Krantz et al. 1991; LaVeau et al. 1989). Burg and colleagues (1993) demonstrated that CAD patients who develop mental stress-induced silent ventricular dysfunction were more likely to respond to stress with anger than CAD patients without mental stress-induced ischemia. The evidence that mental stress is an important precipitator of myocardial ischemia has important implications for the treatment of patients with CAD. These patients may benefit from interventions that focus on the precipitants of and the psychophysiological response to mental stress.

The Setting of Intensive Care

The stress associated with being a patient in an intensive care or coronary care unit is worth discussing briefly. Patients who have had cardiac surgery, an acute MI, or a serious ischemic event are more susceptible to serious ventricular arrhythmias (Fricchione and Vlay 1986; Kamarck and Jennings 1991). Several authors (Goldstein 1987; Stern 1985) documented the high prevalence of anxiety in patients in these intensive care settings. The increase in the sympathetic tone that coexists with anxiety is the probable mechanism for the increased vulnerability to cardiac arrhythmias seen in these patients (Fricchione and Vlay 1986; Kamarck and Jennings 1991). Therefore, patients in these settings may benefit from interventions to decrease their anxiety, especially if they already have a history of serious ventricular arrhythmias. Strategies for treating anxiety in the intensive care setting are discussed elsewhere (Goldstein 1987; Stern 1985).

Sociocultural Factors and Interpersonal Factors

Work "overload" and life stress have also been studied as psychological factors contributing to the development of CAD (Dorian and Taylor 1984; Matthews 1988). Excessive workload and job responsibility and job dissatisfaction have been shown to enhance coronary risk (Krantz and Durel 1983). Previous reviews of the literature on occupational factors and coronary disease conclude that certain occupations may be related to an increased risk of cardiovascular diseases, independent of traditional risk factors (Krantz et al. 1988; Lacroix 1984; Tyroler et al. 1987). Karasek and colleagues (1981, 1982) proposed a job strain model to describe high-risk occupations. In this model, high job strain is defined as the interaction of very demanding work with few opportunities to control the job situation (low decision latitude).

Evidence in support of the job strain model of coronary risk derives from several cross-sectional and some prospective studies. In a 6-year prospective study of Swedish men, those who had jobs characterized by high demand or low control had a 1.3–1.4 times greater risk of coronary heart disease morbidity (e.g., chest pain, dyspnea, hypertension) compared with men whose jobs were high in level of control or low in level of demand (Karasek et al. 1981). A cross-sectional investigation of the Swedish male work force also revealed that shift work and monotony were associated with excess risk of MI (Alfredsson et al. 1982). Moreover, hectic work *in combination* with variables associated with low decision latitude and/or few possibilities for growth was significantly associated with excess risk of MI (Alfredsson et al. 1982). In a 1-year prospective study, occupational characteristics were related to the reason for hospitalization of 958,096 Swedish subjects ages 20–64 years (Alfredsson et al. 1985). Results show that male subjects employed in jobs characterized by the combination of hectic work and few possibilities for growth were more frequently hospitalized for MI than other men (relative risk = 1.6). For women, the combination of hectic and monotonous work conferred greater risk of hospitalization (relative risk = 1.6).

Studies of the United States population have also supported the job strain model of cardiovascular risk. Cross-sectional studies of representative population samples, including the U.S. Health and Education Survey and the National Health and Nutrition Examination Survey, have shown that MI is more prevalent among workers who report high job strain, independent of the influence of traditional risk factors (Karasek et al. 1982). Data from the Framingham study also support the job strain model. Lacroix and Haynes (1987) classified occupational titles for 900 men and women according to job strain. Subjects also rated their level of strain. For both men and women, high-strain job classification was associated with approximately 1.5 times greater risk of coronary heart disease over a 10-year period compared with low-strain classification. Self-ratings of strain, however, conferred even greater risk than objective job classifications for female clerical workers and women in high-strain jobs.

Johnson and Hall (1988) investigated the relationship among job strain, workplace social support, and cardiovascular disease in a cross-sectional sample of 13,779 Swedish male and female workers. They noted that the combination of high job demands, low control, and low social support produced the greatest risk for cardiovascular disease. Research has also shown that employed women with three or more children are twice as likely to develop coronary heart disease as working women with no children. This is especially true for clerical workers who have less help with child care (Haynes et al. 1980). Thus, it appears that job strain affects the risk for cardiovascular disease, and low levels of social support may compound this risk.

A prospective study of the psychosocial influences on mortality after MI was undertaken in 2,320 men who participated in the Beta-Blocker

Heart Attack Trial (Ruberman et al. 1984). When other important prognostic factors were controlled for, patients classified with a high degree of life stress had significantly greater 3-year mortality after an MI than individuals with low life stress. In addition, the presence of the combination of high life stress and high social isolation produced more than four times the risk of death at 3-year follow-up than low levels of stress and isolation. High levels of stress and social isolation were most prevalent among the least-educated men (Ruberman et al. 1984).

Other studies of the relationship between social support and coronary heart disease have found significant, although inconsistent, relationships (Berkman 1985). In the Israeli Ischemic Heart Disease Study, which prospectively followed a cohort of 10,000 adult male Israeli civil service employees, family problems and the lack of spousal support were important predictors of the development of angina pectoris over a 5-year period (Medalie and Goldbourt 1976). There was no relationship between social support and the incidence of MI in the Israeli study (Medalie and Goldbourt 1976), and other prospective studies have not shown a significant relationship between social support and incidence of CAD (Berkman 1985). However, more recently, prospective studies have shown relationships between measures of social support attachment and social integration with coronary heart disease morbidity and mortality (Gorkin et al. 1993; Orth-Gomér et al. 1993).

The relationship between social support and TABP has been the focus of some research (Blumenthal et al. 1987; Orth-Gomér and Unden 1990). In a study of patients undergoing coronary angiography, Blumenthal and colleagues found that Type A subjects with low levels of social support had more severe CAD than Type A subjects with high levels of social support; this relationship was not present for Type B subjects. In a 10-year prospective study of 150 middle-aged Swedish men, lack of social support/social isolation was an independent mortality predictor in Type A men, but not Type B men (Orth-Gomér and Unden 1990). This suggests that social support may have a protective effect in those with TABP.

Our review of sociocultural and interpersonal factors contributing to the development of cardiovascular disease has identified evidence for a positive association among the following factors and CAD: occupational factors (e.g., job strain, low control, few possibilities for growth, low social support at work), life stress, and social isolation. Moreover, social support appears to mitigate the effect of other psychosocial risk factors on cardiovascular disease endpoints.

Investigators have developed an agenda for further research in this area (Tyroler et al. 1987). High on their agenda were studies to assess environmental and psychosocial variables related to CAD risk among individuals with low socioeconomic status. Research to identify and test the efficacy of interventions to increase social support after the development of clinical CAD was also recommended (Tyroler et al. 1987). Studies to test the effect of interventions in the workplace to decrease job strain and increase worker control and social support would also be of great value.

Hypertension

We now review the literature assessing the relationship among psychological and behavioral factors and hypertension. Shapiro (1988) described two categories of psychological factors affecting hypertension: pressor reactivity and personality or behavioral factors.

Physiological Hyperreactivity to Environmental Stimuli: Pressor Reactivity

Several authors reviewed the literature on blood pressure reactivity to experimental and real life stressors and came to similar conclusions (Herd et al. 1987; Houston 1986; Light 1987; Manuck and Krantz 1986; Pickering and Gerin 1988; Shapiro 1988; Weder and Julius 1985). First, there is evidence that there are subsets of individuals that have greater blood pressure reactivity than others to a wide variety of stressors. Second, the evidence linking reactivity in normotensive individuals with the eventual development of hypertension is still somewhat equivocal. The strongest evidence that reactivity may reflect an individual's susceptibility to developing hypertension comes from studies comparing reactivity in normotensive subjects with and without a family history of hypertension. The great majority of these studies found that subjects with a family history of hypertension had greater reactivity than those without a family history (Shapiro 1988). However, in a sample of young black men, this relationship was not found (Anderson et al. 1987). Third, pressor reactivity in patients who have already developed hypertension may exacerbate and even accelerate the disease process (Shapiro 1988). This last conclusion has implications for clinical intervention, because interventions that decrease reactivity or allow the individual to modify stressors may affect the course of the disease process.

Personality or Coping Style

Anger coping styles, interpersonal conflicts, anxiety, and environmental stimuli may all be stressors that produce pressor reactivity or hypertension (Houston 1986; Light 1987; Shapiro 1988). However, almost all of the research is retrospective or cross-sectional in design. The most consistently positive results have involved anger coping styles, but, as noted by Light, studies have found a positive relationship between hypertension and *both* inhibited anger expression and excessive anger expression. Although the associations between suppressed hostility and hypertension are based on retrospective or cross-sectional studies, Dimsdale (1988) pointed out that the strength of the relationship is quite substantial and parallels the relationship between blood pressure and such variables as age, obesity, and social class.

Other investigators have found that individuals who use an active coping style under environmental conditions that are not conducive to success may be predisposed to hypertension (James 1987). Data supporting this concept are derived from reactivity studies that assessed active coping with behavioral stressors that are difficult to control, studies that measured active coping in association with low education and socioeconomic status, and studies that measured high blood pressure in modernizing Third World populations where material aspirations are often discordant with resources (James 1987).

Again, the results of the research in this area have important clinical implications; they suggest the hypothesis that psychological or behavioral treatments to improve anger management or modify coping may lead to improvement in blood pressure control. However, to our knowledge, studies to test this specific hypothesis have not yet been published. However, the efficacy of generic behavioral interventions in the treatment of hypertension have been tested in a number of studies.

Behavioral and Psychological Treatment

The evidence described above, which has linked pressor reactivity and psychological and behavioral factors to the pathogenesis of hypertension, has led investigators to the clinical arena where they have studied the effectiveness of interventions to modify these potential contributing factors and to improve blood pressure control.

Behavioral and psychological treatments of hypertension include psychotherapy, relaxation, and biofeedback. Shapiro (1988) and Chesney and colleagues (1987) also suggested adding placebo, suggestion, and behavioral change (e.g., dietary change, weight loss, smoking cessation, exercise) to the list of behavioral treatments. These treatments are not considered in this review; for a discussion of these approaches, the reader is referred elsewhere (Abrams et al. 1987; Chesney et al. 1987).

The effects of psychotherapy, relaxation, and biofeedback on blood pressure in hypertensive subjects are modest, and thus far there has been little evidence to suggest that sustained effects occur after treatment has been discontinued (Chesney et al. 1987; Shapiro 1988). A meta-analysis of 26 published trials of cognitive or behavioral interventions that met stringent methodological criteria found that these techniques were superior to no therapy, but not superior to credible sham techniques or self-monitoring alone (Eisenberg et al. 1993). Jacob and colleagues (1986) found that although relaxation training could decrease blood pressure among hypertensive patients in the laboratory, there was no significant carryover of the effect into real life when 24-hour ambulatory blood pressure recordings were obtained. Moreover, the effects of medication were significantly greater than the relaxation treatment (Jacob et al. 1986). However, Patel and colleagues (1985) demonstrated that repeated relaxation training has a significant and persistent effect on blood pressure, even after 4 years. These results must be interpreted with caution because 24-hour ambulatory recordings of blood pressure, which has become the preferred measure of blood pressure control (Pickering 1987; Pickering and Gerin 1988), were not obtained as an outcome measure. Another study (Southam et al. 1982), which used 24-hour monitoring of blood pressure, showed that the combination of relaxation therapy and medication was more effective in achieving blood pressure control than a control condition (medication alone); these investigators also demonstrated that the effects of relaxation training were maintained 15 months after treatment (Agras et al. 1983). Glasgow and colleagues (1989) reported the results of a standardized, behavioral stepped-care treatment for hypertension that featured the use of blood pressure monitoring followed by self-administered systolic blood pressure biofeedback and relaxation, in sequence, as needed. All subjects in the behavioral stepped-care and usual-care groups were maintained on pharmacologic agents that were reduced when possible according to a standard protocol. Results demonstrated that the behavioral stepped-care group's medication requirements decreased to levels significantly lower than the usual-care group (Glasgow et al. 1989).

From the studies reviewed, it appears that behavioral procedures are effective in reducing blood pressure and provide additive benefit when combined with pharmacologic treatment. The results of a recent meta-analysis suggest that cognitive and behavioral strategies have limited usefulness, especially when compared with pharmacologic interventions (Eisenberg et al. 1993). However, behavioral interventions may permit reduction in medication dose, although it appears that biofeedback adds little to the practice of relaxation (Chesney et al. 1987). Future studies should assess the effect of behavioral treatment on greater numbers of patients, using 24-hour, ambulatory blood pressure monitoring as an outcome measure and longer follow-up intervals. The combination of behavioral strategies, life-style modification (e.g., dietary change, exercise), and pharmacologic interventions for selected groups of patients also deserves increased attention in future research (Chesney et al. 1987; Eisenberg et al. 1993). Because previous studies have tested the efficacy of behavioral interventions on heterogeneous groups of hypertensive patients, another important research issue is to identify the subgroups that are most likely to respond to specific behavioral treatments. Additionally, studies are needed to develop and test interventions to modify specific behavioral or psychological factors believed to contribute to or exacerbate hypertension (e.g., hostility, anxiety, active coping) in individuals with these characteristics.

Discussion

This chapter and the previous chapter have focused on the extensive literature that explores the relationship between psychological and behavioral factors and cardiovascular disease. For each of the factors listed in Table 2–1 (Chapter 2, this volume), there is sufficient evidence to confirm a relationship. Several summary points can be drawn from the results of this literature review.

First, epidemiologic evidence suggests that the personality construct TABP is a risk factor for the *development* of CAD. However, recent evidence suggests that once CAD is present or risk is high, the presence of global TABP does not increase the risk of having subsequent morbid events, except perhaps sudden cardiac death. Well-controlled studies strongly suggest, however, that subcomponents of TABP (expressive hostility and antagonistic interactions, in particular) predict CAD morbidity and mortality, and aspects of hostility are the subcomponents of TABP that are most related to risk of CAD. Evidence linking TABP and its subcomponents to cardiovascular reactivity provides further indirect evidence of the relationship between these constructs and CAD (see Goldstein and Niaura, Chapter 2, this volume, Figure 2–1). Moreover, although the findings must be considered preliminary, psychological treatment of TABP may improve clinical outcome of CAD.

Despite these positive results, we must not be too hasty in concluding that a cause-and-effect relationship has been demonstrated. Even when a well-controlled prospective investigation produces positive results, these results cannot be taken as evidence for a causal relationship. For example, although hostility may predict cardiovascular morbidity and mortality, it may itself be correlated with some unknown underlying factors (e.g., constitutional trait, environmental or situational factors) that simultaneously promote both hostility and the disease process. Note again that the arrows in Figure 2–1 (Goldstein and Niaura, Chapter 2, this volume) between TABP and cardiovascular reactivity go both ways. Moreover, as social learning theory suggests (Price 1982), the consequences of behavior, including the development of illness and morbid events, influence the expression of subsequent behavior. Although the evidence suggests that treatments targeted to reduce aspects of TABP reduce cardiovascular risk, these treatments are likely to be most effective for subgroups of individuals (e.g., those with higher levels of social support). Future research needs to address this issue. Research is also needed to determine which constellation of psychosocial factors predict response to psychosocial interventions. For example, do men and women (and white versus nonwhite; low education versus high education) respond to psychosocial treatments differently?

Second, there is evidence that patients with a major depressive disorder are at increased risk for a cardiovascular morbidity and mortality, although the evidence linking depressive symptoms and CAD is not consistent.

Third, there is little evidence to suggest a significant relationship between patient anxiety and CAD outcomes because research in this area has not been methodologically sound. However, there is considerable evidence linking disturbing situations and life events with myocardial ischemia, ventricular arrhythmias, and sudden death. The model described by Kamarck and Jennings (1991) to delineate the pathways of psychological influences in sudden death (see Figure 3–1) is useful for understanding the mechanism by which psychological factors influence a specific cardiac endpoint. This model also provides a blueprint for future research in this area, as described earlier. Research must focus more on identifying the biological mechanisms that mediate the relationship between psychological and behavioral factors and disease endpoints. For example, there should be increased attention paid to the effects of psychological factors on the activity of the sympathoadrenal and hypothalamic-pituitary-adrenocortical axes.

Fourth, occupational factors such as high job strain, low control, and few possibilities for growth are significantly associated with excess risk of CAD.

Fifth, low levels of social support appear to interact with life stress, job strain, and TABP to increase risk for CAD events. Although more large-scale prospective studies of the relationship of sociodemographic and psychobehavioral factors with cardiovascular disease would be helpful, researchers must pay more attention to interactions among risk factors rather than relying on partitioning strategies to isolate the variables in which the investigators are interested at the time of the study. We must simultaneously pay attention to those sociobehavioral factors (e.g., poverty, race, diet, smoking, social support) that we know are related to cardiovascular risk but are also related to psychological constructs such as hostility. Research must address this level of complexity in design, measurement, and analysis.

Finally, with respect to hypertension, there is considerable evidence that suggests pressor reactivity is a risk factor for the development of hypertension and some evidence to suggest that pressor reactivity is a risk factor for the progression of this disease. There is also evidence linking personality or coping style with both pressor reactivity and hypertension, but almost all the research is retrospective or cross-sectional in design. The relationship between psychological factors and the maintenance of hypertension is indirectly supported by evidence demonstrating the effects of behavioral interventions on blood pressure.

References

Abrams DB, Raciti MA, Ruggiero L, et al: Cardiovascular risk factor reduction in the medical setting, in Principles of Medical Psychiatry. Edited by Stoudemire A, Fogel BS. Orlando, FL, Grune & Stratton, 1987, pp 347–363

Agras WS, Southam MA, Taylor CB: Long-term persistence of relaxation-induced blood pressure lowering during the working day. J Consult Clin Psychol 51:792–794, 1983

Alfredsson L, Karasek R, Theorell T: Myocardial infarction and psychosocial work environment: an analysis of the male Swedish working force. Soc Sci Med 16:463–467, 1982

Alfredsson L, Spetz CL, Theorell T: Type of occupation and near-future hospitalization for myocardial infarction and some other diagnoses. Int J Epidemiol 14:378–388, 1985

Anderson NB, Williams RB Jr, Lane JD, et al: Parental history of hypertension and cardiovascular responses to behavioral stress in young black men. J Psychosom Res 31:723–729, 1987

Berkman LF: The relationship of social networks and social support to morbidity and mortality, in Social Support and Health. Edited by Cohen S, Syme SL. Orlando, FL, Academic Press, 1985, pp 241–262

Blumenthal JA, Burg MM, Barefoot J, et al: Social support, Type A behavior, and coronary artery disease. Psychosom Med 49:331–340, 1987

Burg MM, Jain D, Soufer R, et al: Role of behavioral and psychological factors in mental stress-induced silent left ventricular dysfunction in coronary artery disease. J Am Coll Cardiol 22:440–448, 1993

Chesney MA, Agras WA, Benson H, et al: Nonpharmacologic approaches to the treatment of hypertension. Circulation 76 (suppl I):I-104–I-109, 1987

Deanfield JE, Kensett M, Wilson RA, et al: Silent myocardial ischemia due to mental stress. Lancet 2:1001–1004, 1984

Dimsdale JE: Research links between psychiatry and cardiology: hypertension, Type A behavior, sudden death, and the physiology of emotional arousal. Gen Hosp Psychiatry 10:328–338, 1988

Dimsdale JE, Ruberman W, Carleton RA, et al: Sudden cardiac death: stress and cardiac arrhythmias. Circulation 76 (suppl I):I-198–I-201, 1987

Dorian B, Taylor CB: Stress factors in the development of coronary artery disease. J Occup Med 26:747–756, 1984

Eisenberg DM, Delbanco TL, Berkey CS, et al: Cognitive behavioral techniques for hypertension: are they effective? Ann Intern Med 118:964–972, 1993

Epstein SE, Quyyumi AA, Bonow RO: Myocardial ischemia: silent or symptomatic. N Engl J Med 318:1038–1043, 1988

Follick MJ, Gorkin L, Capone RJ, et al: Psychological distress as a predictor of ventricular arrhythmias in a post-myocardial infarct population. Am Heart J 116:32–36, 1988

Follick MJ, Ahern DK, Gorkin L, et al: Relation of psychosocial and stress reactivity variables to ventricular arrhythmias in the Cardiac Arrhythmia Pilot Study (CAPS). Am J Cardiol 66:63–67, 1990

Fricchione GL, Vlay SC: Psychiatric aspects of patients with malignant ventricular arrhythmias. Am J Psychiatry 143:1518–1526, 1986

Glasgow MS, Engel BT, D'Lugoff BC: A controlled trial of a standardized behavioral stepped treatment for hypertension. Psychosom Med 51:10–26, 1989

Goldstein MG: Intensive care unit syndromes, in Principles of Medical Psychiatry. Edited by Stoudemire A, Fogel B. Orlando, FL, Grune & Stratton, 1987, pp 403–421

Gorkin L, Schron EB, Brooks MM, et al: Psychosocial predictors of mortality in the Cardiac Arrhythmia Suppression Trial-1 (CAST-1). Am J Cardiol 71:263–267, 1993

Greene W, Goldstein S, Moss A: Psychosocial aspects of sudden death. Arch Intern Med 129:725–731, 1972

Haynes SG, Feinleib M, Kannel WB: The relationship of psychosocial factors to coronary heart disease in the Framingham Study, III: eight-year incidence of coronary heart disease. Am J Epidemiol 111:37–58, 1980

Herd JA, Falkner O, Anderson DE, et al: Psychophysiologic factors in hypertension. Circulation 76 (suppl I):I-89–I-94, 1987

Houston BK: Psychological variables and cardiovascular and neuroendocrine reactivity, in Handbook of Stress, Reactivity, and Cardiovascular Disease. Edited by Matthews KA, Weiss SM, Detre T, et al. New York, Wiley, 1986, pp 207–229

Jacob RG, Shapiro AP, Reeves RA, et al: Comparison of relaxation therapy for hypertension with placebo, diuretics and beta-blockers. Arch Intern Med 146:2335–2340, 1986

James SA: Psychosocial precursors of hypertension: a review of the epidemiologic evidence. Circulation 76 (suppl I):I-60–I-66, 1987

Johnson JV, Hall EM: Job strain, work place social support, and cardiovascular disease: a cross-sectional study of a random sample of the Swedish working population. Am J Public Health 78:1336–1342, 1988

Kamarck T, Jennings JR: Biobehavioral factors in sudden cardiac death. Psychol Bull 109:42–75, 1991

Karasek R, Baker D, Marxer F, et al: Job decision latitude, job demands, and cardiovascular disease: a prospective study of Swedish men. Am J Public Health 71:694–705, 1981

Karasek RA, Theorell TG, Schwartz J, et al: Job, psychological factors, and coronary heart disease: Swedish prospective findings and U.S. prevalence findings using a new occupational inference method. Adv Cardiol 29:62–87, 1982

Krantz DS, Durel LA: Psychobiological substrates of the Type A behavior pattern. Health Psychol 2:393–411, 1983

Krantz DS, Contrada RJ, Hill DR, et al: Environmental stress and biobehavioral antecedents of coronary heart disease. J Consult Clin Psychol 56:333–341, 1988

Krantz DS, Helmers KF, Bairey CN, et al: Cardiovascular reactivity and mental stress-induced myocardial ischemia in patients with coronary artery disease. Psychosom Med 53:1–12, 1991

Lacroix AZ: Occupational exposure to high demand/low control work and coronary heart disease incidence in the Framingham cohort. Unpublished doctoral dissertation, University of North Carolina at Chapel Hill, 1984

Lacroix AZ, Haynes SG: Gender differences in the stressfulness of workplace roles: a focus on work and health, in Gender and Stress. Edited by Barnett E, Baruch G, Biener L. New York, Free Press, 1987, pp 96–121

LaVeau PJ, Rozanski A, Krantz DS, et al: Transient left ventricular dysfunction during provocative mental stress in patients with coronary artery disease. Am Heart J 118:1–8, 1989

Light KC: Psychosocial precursors of hypertension: experimental evidence. Circulation 76 (suppl I):I-67–I-76, 1987

Lown B: Sudden cardiac death: biobehavioral perspective. Circulation 76 (suppl I):I-186–I-196, 1987

Lown B, DeSilva RA: Roles of psychologic stress and autonomic nervous system changes in provocation of ventricular premature complexes. Am J Cardiol 41:979–985, 1978

Matthews KA: Coronary heart disease and Type A behaviors: update on and alternative to the Booth-Kewley and Friedman (1987) quantitative review. Psychol Bull 104:373–380, 1988

Manuck SB, Krantz DW: Psychophysiologic reactivity in coronary heart disease and essential hypertension, in Handbook of Stress, Reactivity, and Cardiovascular Disease. Edited by Matthews KA, Weiss SM, Detre T, et al. New York, John Wiley, 1986, pp 11–34

Medalie J, Goldbourt V: Angina pectoris among 10,000 men, II: psychosocial and other risk factors as evidenced by a multivariate analyses of a five-year incidence study. Am J Med 60:910–921, 1976

Myers A, Dewar N: Circumstances attending 100 sudden deaths from coronary artery disease with coroner's necropsies. Br Heart J 37:1133–1143, 1975

Orth-Gomér K, Unden AL: Type A behavior, social support, and coronary risk: interaction and significance for mortality in cardiac patients. Psychosom Med 52:59–72, 1990

Orth-Gomér K, Rosengren A, Wilhelmsen L: Lack of social support and incidence of coronary heart disease in middle-aged Swedish men. Psychosom Med 55:37–43, 1993

Patel C, Marmot MG, Terry DJ, et al: Trial of relaxation in reducing coronary risk: four year follow-up. BMJ 290:1102–1106, 1985

Pickering TG: Strategies for the evaluation and treatment of hypertension and some implications of blood pressure variability. Circulation 76 (suppl I):I-77–I-82, 1987

Pickering TG, Gerin W: Ambulatory blood pressure monitoring and cardiovascular reactivity for the evaluation of the role of psychosocial factors and prognosis in hypertensive patients. Am Heart J 116:665–672, 1988

Price VA: Type A Behavior Pattern: A Model for Research and Practice. New York, Academic Press, 1982

Reich P, DeSilva RA, Lown B, et al: Acute psychological disturbance preceding life-threatening ventricular arrhythmias. JAMA 246:233–235, 1981

Rozanski A, Bairey CN, Krantz DS, et al: Mental stress and the induction of silent myocardial ischemia in patients with coronary artery disease. N Engl J Med 318:1005–1012, 1988

Ruberman W, Weinblatt E, Goldberg JD, et al: Psychological influences on mortality after myocardial infarction. N Engl J Med 311:552–559, 1984

Schwartz PJ: Stress and sudden cardiac death: the role of the autonomic nervous system. Journal of Clinical Psychiatry Monograph Series 2:7–13, 1984

Schwartz PJ, La Rovere MT, Vanoli E: Autonomic nervous system and sudden cardiac death: experimental basis and clinical observations for post-myocardial infarction risk stratification. Circulation 85 (suppl I):I-77–I-91, 1992

Selwyn AP, Ganz P: Myocardial ischemia in coronary disease. N Engl J Med 318:1058–1060, 1988

Shapiro AP: Psychological factors in hypertension: an overview. Am Heart J 116:632–637, 1988

Siltanen P: Life changes and sudden coronary death. Adv Cardiol 25:47–60, 1978

Southam MA, Agras WS, Taylor CB, et al: Relaxation training: blood pressure reduction during the working day. Arch Gen Psychiatry 39:715–717, 1982

Stern TA: The management of depression and anxiety following myocardial infarction. Mt Sinai J Med 52:623–633, 1985

Tavazzi L, Zotti AM, Rondanelli R: The role of psychologic stress in the genesis of lethal arrhythmias in patients with coronary artery disease. Eur Heart J 7 (suppl A):99–106, 1986

Tyroler A, Haynes SG, Cobb LA, et al: Environmental risk factors in coronary heart disease. Circulation 76 (suppl I):I-139–I-144, 1987

Weder AB, Julius S: Behavior, blood pressure variability, and hypertension. Psychosom Med 47:406–414, 1985

CHAPTER 4

Neurological Conditions

Depression and Stroke, Multiple Sclerosis, Parkinson's Disease, and Epilepsy

M. EILEEN MCNAMARA, M.D.

Psychiatry has played an important part in drawing attention to the significant role mental processes play in the presentation of physical illness. Current research in psychoimmunology, psychoendocrinology, and a number of other areas has antecedents in the work of many early investigators of psychosomatic illness. Both Franz Alexander and Adolph Meyer, as well as other founders of psychosomatic medicine, established that patients' symptoms have multiple etiologies with varying contributions of psychological and nonpsychological causes.

For these pioneers, the term *psychosomatic* was not meant to imply a single cause of an illness, but rather an approach to the patient that included both mental and physical factors. The elegance of this approach was overlooked by many later clinicians, who tended to divide illnesses into "functional" versus "organic" disorders.

The category psychological factors affecting physical condition was introduced into DSM-III (American Psychiatric Association 1980) in a partial effort to restore the intent of these early investigators. The explicit intention was to avoid simplistic, unimodal statements about causality,

---

This chapter is dedicated to the memory of Dr. John Neil.

but also to allow the recognition that psychological factors can play a role in the initiation, exacerbation, or maintenance of a disease.

For some illnesses, these connections seem fairly straightforward. The definition of psychological factors affecting neurological disorders, however, entails some difficult etiologic questions. Unless a strictly Cartesian viewpoint is maintained, it is difficult to make causal connections between psychiatric and neurological disorders because it is uncertain whether two "separate," interacting processes are involved, or just two aspects of one unified brain process. By accepting the provisional concept of psychological and neurological factors being "associated" rather than causally related, a safer terminology is employed. The methodology used to investigate the relationships between psychological and neurological illness, however, is predicated on concepts involving the definition and relationship of these two categories.

In this chapter, as a contribution to the revision of the DSM-III-R (American Psychiatric Association 1987) category psychological factors affecting physical condition for DSM-IV (American Psychiatric Association 1994), I attempt to deduce and make explicit these assumptions and to note the way that these concepts have evolved over time from early Cartesian viewpoints to more recent deterministic models of human behavior. The delineation of these relationships is of more than just philosophical interest; the acceptance of these models has implications for etiology and treatment as well. In the following review, I summarize psychiatry's understanding of how psychiatric illness is related to four major neurological disorders: stroke, multiple sclerosis, Parkinson's disease, and epilepsy. Because these disorders cover a spectrum of possible psychiatric symptoms, I focus primarily on depression and its relationship to these neurological disorders.

An attempt was made in this review to include examples of major studies in this century from the psychiatric and neurological literature. Criteria for inclusion varied somewhat with the decade of the research since research and methodological standards have evolved significantly over the years. A detailed critique of each study was not possible, however, in a chapter of this length. Moreover, since standards of diagnosis both for psychiatric and neurological illness have undergone considerable refinement over the years, conclusions reached in prior years at times have become problematic. As an example, Pond and Bidwell

(1959) reported that 38% of epileptic patients had some form of psychiatric illness. With modern diagnostic investigation, however, almost certainly a portion of those patients would be found today to have hypothyroidism, subdural hematomas, meningiomas, or other illnesses underlying their mental symptoms. Indeed, today not only might these patients not be thought to have psychiatric illness, it is likely that closed-circuit telemetry electroencephalogram or depth electrodes would show that a significant number of them do not even have epilepsy. With these considerations in mind, the first disorder reviewed is that of stroke and depression.

Stroke

Kraepelin (1901/1915) first noted that patients with cerebrovascular disease were vulnerable to depression. Early investigators tended to view such depression as an understandable reaction to brain injury (Benson 1973; Charatan and Fish 1978; Geschwind 1970). Such a view is not unreasonable given the abrupt and profound changes in functional ability and social roles that a stroke often entails.

Initial research examined the way that a variety of social and psychological factors influence the outcome of rehabilitation; in general, this research suggested that a high level of self-esteem improves the outcome of patients (Barry et al. 1968; Cogswell 1968; MacGuiffe et al. 1969; Slater et al. 1970). Hyman (1972a), for example, examined 110 patients in a stroke rehabilitation center using rating scales to assess attitudes toward present life-style and illness and self-image, comparing these against ratings of motivation and improvement. This study was limited to patients who were sufficiently cognitively intact (thereby excluding patients with significant dominant hemisphere strokes and aphasia). Feelings of stigma and social isolation among these patients and dissatisfaction with family life correlated with poor motivation and less functional improvement.

Implicit in most of the earlier work was the assumption that psychological characteristics are separate and independently mutable from the effects of the stroke itself. This position was gradually challenged. Folstein and colleagues (1977) compared 20 stroke and orthopedic patients who were equally functionally disabled, using the Hamilton Rating Scale for Depression (HRSD) and the Present State Examination. He found that 45% of the stroke patients had evidence of depression as compared with 10% of the orthopedic patients, failing therefore to support the hypothesis that depression was a simple reaction to functional disability.

During the same period, the field of psychiatry in general was making a conceptual turn away from looking at separate psychological traits toward examining psychiatric illnesses with explicit criteria. For example, many of Hyman's (1972a) patients with feelings of isolation and unhappiness today might be considered to have major depression. Robinson and colleagues (1983, 1984) published a large series of studies on the relationship between stroke and depression. In 1982, Robinson and Price reported a series of 103 patients admitted for stroke and followed through rehabilitation. Defining depression by DSM-III criteria, he reported a 26% incidence of depression and a 20% incidence of dysthymia at the time of the stroke. After 6 months, the prevalence of depression had increased to 34%, and the prevalence of dysthymia had increased to 26%. In other words, only 40% of stroke patients did not become depressed. These depressions tended to be significant and long-lasting when treated. Furthermore, the presence of such depression appeared to have a direct impact on the degree of functional recovery. The presence of depression in these patients was independently predictive of poorer social functioning. In this 2-year longitudinal study, the severity of depression did not correlate with the severity of neurological impairment. On the other hand, severity of depression did correlate with impairment of functional ability. Initially, depression accounted for only 10% of the variance, whereas lesion location accounted for 50%. At 6 months, however, there was an increase in the association between functional impairment and depression, with a correlation coefficient of .65.

In 1986, Robinson and colleagues reported a series of 38 patients with a left hemisphere stroke. Patients were evaluated with the Zung Self-Rating Depression Scale, the HRSD, the Present State Examination, the Johns Hopkins Functioning Inventory, and the Mini-Mental State Exam (MMSE). Psychiatric diagnoses were assigned by DSM-III criteria. Among the nondepressed patients, the severity of intellectual impairment was related to lesion location and volume, as expected. The depressed patients, however, showed more cognitive impairment than expected by lesion volume alone. All patients with major depression showed some degree of cognitive impairment, whereas only 40% of nondepressed patients displayed such impairment. More significantly, although the nondepressed patients demonstrated some cognitive improvement at 6-month follow-up, the depressed patients showed no such improvement. The authors also anecdotally noted their observation that cognitive function improved when depression was successfully treated.

In 1989, Bolla-Wilson and colleagues repeated this study, dividing patients into left versus right hemisphere stroke. Patients with aphasia were excluded from the study. Patients in this study were subjected to a much more detailed battery of neuropsychological tests and were rated for depression with the Zung and Hamilton depression scales and the Present State Examination. Patients were also given the MMSE. Those with left hemisphere strokes with depression did significantly worse on cognitive tests than those who were not depressed. Right hemisphere stroke did not produce this effect because both depressed and nondepressed patients had similar scores on the MMSE.

It remains unclear, however, why some but not all patients develop depression. Robinson and Starkstein (1990) emphasized the role of subcortical atrophy and family history of affective disorders in the vulnerability to poststroke depression.

Using positron-emission tomography, Mayberg and colleagues (1988) showed alterations in serotonin receptor binding following stroke that paralleled the severity of the depression. This suggests that poststroke depression has neurochemical, not just neuroanatomical, underpinnings, and it suggests that the depression might respond to pharmacological maneuvers. There is still, however, only a small body of work about the pharmacological treatment of poststroke depression and about the effects of successful treatment. Reding (1986), using trazodone, and Lipsey and colleagues (1985), using nortriptyline, reported successful treatment of a small percentage of poststroke depression, but with a high incidence of side effects. For patients who could be successfully treated, Reding reported a consistent trend toward improvement in activities of daily living scores; Lipsey and colleagues could not show any functional improvement compared with placebo.

Multiple Sclerosis

An interesting example of conceptual turns in neuropsychiatry is that euphoria, until fairly recently, was thought to be a cardinal symptom of multiple sclerosis (MS); now depression is considered the chief psychiatric implication of MS. S. Brown and Davis (1922), for example, reported that 90% of MS patients had "mental alterations" and that euphoria was present in 71%. Cottrell and Wilson (1926) examined 100 consecutive patients and reported that 63% had euphoria, 10% had depression, and 23% had labile mood. Just prior to computed tomography, euphoria was considered a strong diagnostic clue to the presence of MS.

The apparent disappearance of these once-prominent symptoms is probably attributable to changes in the definition of both MS and of euphoria. MS is protean in its diverse presentation. Despite improvements in neuroimaging, immunological assays, and electrodiagnostics, there is still no simple or entirely reliable way to make an antemortem diagnosis of MS. Thus, it is probable that many of the patients reported earlier in the century had other illnesses, such as neurosyphilis, collagen vascular disease, and so forth. Wechsler (1921), for example, reported a survey of 1,773 MS patients and included in his group patients with "infantile, congenital, familial, and hereditary" forms of MS. Although he reported a 9% incidence of euphoria and a 12% incidence of depression, it is virtually certain that some of these patients now would be considered to have some illness other than MS.

Moreover, what was once considered the psychological symptom of euphoria would now probably be reclassified as the neurological symptom of frontal lobe disinhibition. Because the demyelinating lesions of MS tend to be periventricular, they may preferentially disconnect connecting fibers of the frontal lobe and produce disinhibition, lack of concern, and poor judgment. Although mania, which can have euphoria as a symptom, has been reported by Schiffer and colleagues (1986) to be twice as common as expected in MS, no author has reported the huge incidence of euphoria that would substantiate what investigators reported earlier in this century.

As opposed to the de-emphasis of euphoria, there has been an increasing focus of attention on depression in MS. As noted above, early research documented an association between MS and depression, but the association was minor and infrequent. Braceland and Giffen (1950) reported that 20% of MS patients were depressed, consistent with the prevalence of 18% reported by Kahana and colleagues (1971). Depression, when present, was thought to be a psychological reaction to physical disability. Surridge (1969) performed the first controlled study of psychiatric changes in MS, with psychiatric diagnosis assigned by clinical interview. He found no significant differences in the incidence of depressive symptoms in 108 MS patients (27%, compared to a 13% depression rate among 39 control subjects with muscular dystrophy), and he concluded that the majority of depressed MS patients were suffering from reactive illness. In 1980, however, Whitlock and Siskind compared 30 MS patients with 30 patients with other neurological illnesses. Patients with MS were significantly more depressed at interview than the patients with equal disability from other neurological illnesses; 16 of the 30 MS patients and 5 of the 30 control subjects were felt to have an "endogenous" depression. Although for both groups the degree of depression correlated in a limited way with the degree of disability, disability alone did not explain the depression. Interestingly, eight of the MS patients, but none of the control subjects, reported the onset of depression before the onset of neurological illness. Clearly, in this group, depression could not be associated with a neurological illness that did not yet exist. The authors concluded that serious affective illness could be a premonitory symptom of MS or a later complication of the disease. Subsequently, further studies were undertaken to approach this issue in a more rigorous fashion.

In 1983, Schiffer and colleagues reported 15 patients with predominantly cerebral MS matched to 15 patients with predominantly spinal MS and 15 control subjects. Significantly, 9 of the 15 patients in the cerebral MS group reported 11 prior depressive episodes, whereas only 2 patients in the noncerebral MS group had experienced one episode each. The patients in this study tended to interpret their depressive episodes as psychological reactions to stressful events occasioned by the advance of MS. Depressive episodes typically occurred with a flare-up of the MS, or they were associated with a disturbance in an important relationship or work role. The noncerebral group, however, suffered equal functional decline as well as substantial social loss, yet they did not suffer major depression nearly as often.

In 1983, Dalos and colleagues reported on the first prospective study of the relationship between disease activity and affective state in MS. They followed 64 patients for 1 year. Patients completed the 28-item General Health Questionnaire at the time of entry into the study and thereafter on a monthly basis. All patients received a complete neurological examination for which a Kurtzke Disability score was derived. These patients were matched with 23 patients who had static spinal cord injuries, who also completed the General Health Questionnaire on a monthly basis. Dalos and colleagues found that 90% of the patients who had progressive or relapsing MS had emotional disturbance, compared with 39% of the patients with stable MS and 12% of the spinal cord injury group.

Several case reports and surveys have suggested that depression may be the first sign of MS, preceding overt neurological symptoms by months to years (Matthews 1979; Young et al. 1976). Until the introduction of magnetic resonance imaging, it has been impossible to determine the exact onset of MS; to avoid diagnostic doubt, early studies excluded patients of recent onset. In an effort to clarify the relationship among cognitive impairment, depression, neurological symptoms, and disease chronicity, Lyon-Caen and colleagues (1986) examined 30 patients with neurological symptoms of less than 24 months. Of these patients, 11 met criteria for major depression according to DSM-III criteria. The authors also made the important distinction between abnormalities of mood and abnormalities of the expression of affect, such as affective incontinence, lability, and oversensitivity to emotional stimuli. Although in control subjects mood and affect are closely linked, certain neurological lesions can cause a dissociation between felt emotion (mood) and expressed emotion (affect). Pseudobulbar palsy and emotional incontinence are characteristic of MS; a significant limitation of many studies is the neglect of this distinction. With MS, patients may cry without being depressed or laugh without feeling humor. A total of 9 of the 19 nondepressed patients and 5 of the 11 depressed patients had alterations such as pseudobulbar lability, as measured by the Specific Mood Scale. The authors also found a 60% incidence of cognitive impairment in early MS. They found no relationship between the presence of depression and cognitive handicap.

Homer and colleagues (1987) utilized the increased sensitivity of magnetic resonance imaging to examine eight patients with MS and psychiatric problems compared with eight matched MS control patients without psychiatric symptoms. Diagnoses were made by DSM criteria. Seven of the eight subjects had affective disorder, and one had organic hallucinosis. All psychiatric symptoms in these patients had begun at or after the onset of MS but did not correlate consistently with exacerbations. Total lesion area on magnetic resonance imaging was the same for case subjects and control subjects. The case subjects, however, showed significantly more temporal lobe involvement: 488 mm compared with 280 mm for control subjects. No other brain area showed such a difference.

In an intriguing but chiefly impressionistic article, Schiffer (1987) attempted to integrate previous literature and present his view of the nature of depression in MS and provide an approach for clinical management. He interviewed 72 patients referred for depressive symptoms over a 2-year period from a clinic of 430 patients with MS. Patients who appeared moderately or severely depressed also were given the Schedule for Affective Disorders and Schizophrenia (SADS). He added the term *situational* to the Research Diagnostic Criteria (RDC) (Spitzer et al. 1978) to describe those patients whose depressive features arose in the setting of deterioration in neurological status. This vague term implies a particular causal relationship. Patients were assigned ad hoc to biological, social, or psychotherapeutic treatment. The length of treatment (5 weeks) was brief, and the numbers in each group were so small that the results are of uncertain significance. What is interesting, however, is the differences Schiffer observed between depressed patients in whom MS was active and those in whom it was not. Patients who became depressed when their MS was active tended to improve with time, regardless of clinical management. These patients commonly feared loss of independent function. By contrast, patients in whom MS was not active appeared to Schiffer, in some way, to fear getting better. "The inactive group, however, seemed much more comfortable with a socially dependent status, and in 6 of these 7 patients, the depression actually supervened when events augured a need to increase their level of independent function" (p. 599). Schiffer believed that these patients feared the loss of dependent gratification. Although unsystematized, this article introduced an interesting new variable to consider in the potential connections between MS and depression.

Boyle and colleagues (1991) expanded on this when she noted that much research on the psychological problems of MS implies that patients differ in quantity rather than quality of abnormalities. Cluster analysis of Minnesota Multiphasic Personality Inventory scores of 99 MS patients yielded four profiles of psychological problems in MS: depression 14%, denial-euphoria 32%, exaggeration of physical problems 22%, and affective changes consistent with level of disability 31%.

Joffe and colleagues (1987) reported the best study to date of the association of mood disorders with MS. Most previous studies had failed to use standardized psychiatric assessments, defining depression on mood scales without further diagnostic criteria. They studied 100 patients with a modified SADS-Lifetime (SADS-L), assigning RDC diagnoses, and made the diagnosis of psychiatric disorder even more stringent by including the requirement that patients previously must have sought professional help and not just suffered functional impairment. Patients were also given the Beck Depression Inventory, the Present State Anxiety Scale, the Symptom Checklist—90, Revised, the HRSD, the Manic State Rating Scale, and the Kurtzke Functional Disability Scale. The study also introduced the important refinement that the diagnosis of affective disorder be excluded if temporally related to the use of steroids. With all of these rigorous and fairly stringent methods of definition, the authors derived an astounding 72% incidence of psychiatric problems in the MS population. The most common illness was depression (42%). Contrary to some other reports, there was no correlation between functional disability and mood. In fact, the 28 patients without a lifetime psychiatric diagnosis had the highest functional disability.

Although the etiology of mood changes in MS remains in part unknown, and likely is multifactorial, Foley and colleagues (1992) provided evidence of one possible mechanism. In a 2-year prospective study of 22 patients with MS participating in a placebo-controlled trial of cyclosporine, times of greater depression were associated with lower CD8 cell numbers and CD8 percentage and a higher CD4-to-CD8 ratio. It may be that psychological distress or stress serves as one of many triggers that sets into motion the inflammatory and immunological changes characteristic of MS.

Parkinson's Disease

Anyone who ever "shook with fear" or "froze with anxiety" realizes on reflection that mood and motor activity are linked. These links are particularly clear in Parkinson's disease, in which functional activity can change from minute to minute depending on mood state. Early observations tended to take the psychological states of these patients as primary, capable of influencing the course of Parkinson's disease. Many authors had noted a premorbid rigid and inflexible personality style in these patients, the emotional equivalent of the motor impairment. At first, this was thought by some to be the actual cause of Parkinson's disease. As late as 1951, Prichard and colleagues suggested that chronic emotional stress might cause chemical changes in predisposed individuals, resulting in the motor disease. The current view that Parkinson's disease is not caused by psychogenic factors was widely accepted only after 1959, when Riklan and colleagues reported a series of 108 patients carefully studied with a screening interview and neuropsychological test battery. Others continued to study psychological factors, however, for their effects on the progress of the disease. For example, several studies (Prichard et al. 1951; Singer 1976) examined the effect of psychological variables on treatment outcome. Personality traits were inferred from a questionnaire. Prichard and colleagues reported that patients who were dependent and suggestible tended to improve more; on the other hand, Singer found that patients who expected more of themselves did better. These contradictory results may be an effect of the different instruments employed.

Research has focused on the incidence of depression in Parkinson's disease rather than more broadly defined psychological profiles. Depression was first noted by Parkinson himself in his original description of the disease. In initial reports, depression was defined impressionistically, such as in the report by Warburton (1967), who found severe depression in 60% of women and 52% of men referred for thalamotomy. Celesia and Wannamaker (1972) reported a prevalence of 37%. Later authors used standardized rating scales. L. G. Brown and Wilson (1972) reported that 52% of Parkinson's outpatients met criteria for depression as defined by the HRSD. This study was retrospective and assigned diagnosis by chart review. Mindham (1970) reported that depression accounted for 90% of psychiatric hospitalizations of Parkinson's patients.

The disability associated with Parkinson's disease was also initially thought to be the cause of depressive symptoms (Hyman 1972b; Mindham 1970). A number of studies later refuted the idea that depression was simply a reaction to disability by finding a significantly higher incidence in Parkinson's groups than in patients with other disabling illnesses (L. G. Brown and Wilson 1972; Robins 1976; Warburton 1967) and by finding that successful treatment with L-dopa and improvement in functional ability did not necessarily cause improvement in depression (Cherington 1970; Marsh and Markham 1973).

The degree of disability in Parkinson's disease can change quite rapidly, however; Cantello and colleagues (1986) took advantage of this to allow patients to serve as their own control subjects. Parkinson's patients treated with medications may develop significant fluctuations in motor functioning over the course of hours, termed the *on-off phenomena,* a subset of which is the *end-of-dose phenomenon,* which is thought to be due to dropping levels of dopamine. Patients were given a modified Beck Depression Inventory. To separate reactive from primary effects, patients were carefully matched to patients with rheumatoid arthritis who also have periods of greater and less mobility, but for reasons not related to the central nervous system. The authors found that immobility was indeed temporally related to worsening of mood but that such depression was more marked in the Parkinson's patients, suggesting that reactive factors alone could not explain all of the variance.

Although not originally thought to be part of the illness, dementia has been recognized as an important and common complication of Parkinson's disease. Earlier studies did not address the presence or absence of dementia, which could have confounded the results. This was remedied by Mayeux and colleagues (1981) in their study of depression in Parkinson's disease. They reported a series of 55 Parkinson's patients, excluding patients who were overtly demented. Patients were given the Beck Depression Inventory and the MMSE with additional questions to broaden evaluations of language, memory, attention, and praxis. Tasks were not timed, a crucial consideration in evaluating bradykinetic patients. Patients also received a neurological examination, at which time the neurologist completed a Parkinson's disease evaluation form, rating the severity of the symptoms on a scale from 1 to 4.

Mayeux and colleagues (1981) reported that 47% of the Parkinson's patients were depressed. Most of these depressions were mild, but 35% did report that moderate to severe depression began before Parkinson's disease was clinically evident. Mayeux and colleagues also found a correlation between the severity of depression and the impairment of cognitive skills and attention, and they postulated a unifying brain mechanism. Similar results were reported by Santamaria and colleagues (1986).

In 1986, Mayeux and colleagues refined this research by using DSM-III criteria and reported that in 49 consecutive nondemented patients, 28% met criteria for major depression and 14% for dysthymia. Both the National Institute of Mental Health Diagnostic Interview Schedule and the HRSD were used. Depression correlated with lower cerebrospinal fluid 5-hydroxyindoleacetic acid (5-HIAA), suggesting a reduction in central serotonin. Treatment with a serotonin precursor resulted in improvement and in a return of cerebrospinal fluid 5-HIAA levels to normal (Mayeux et al. 1984, 1988).

Schiffer and colleagues (1988) further defined this population by studying 26 patients with Parkinson's disease and depression with the SADS-L, assigning RDC diagnoses. They noticed a fairly high prevalence of anxiety in the depressed patients (12 of 16) and found 8 with panic disorder. In 7 of these 8, panic did not begin until after the onset of neurological symptoms, which is in striking contrast to the usual history of panic disorder, beginning in young adulthood. They suggested that the relatively late onset of anxiety and panic in these patients might link these symptoms to the pathophysiology of Parkinson's disease.

Work by Starkstein and colleagues (1989) suggests that early-onset Parkinson's disease, generally defined as occurring before age 55, may differ in both etiology and phenomenology from late-onset Parkinson's disease. The authors examined the incidence of depression in 105 consecutive patients. Using DSM-III criteria, 37% of the 41 early-onset patients were found to have major depression, and a further 24% were found to have dysthymia. Of the 64 members of the late-onset group, only 10% had major depression, and 17% had dysthymia. This finding of significantly more depression in the younger population stands in marked contrast to the expected higher incidence of depression with age. In the younger patients, depression correlated with cognitive impairments and duration of the disease, although one must question how the effects of depression were separated from the effects of dementia on the MMSE. Only in the older patients did functional impairment correlate with degree of depression, again suggesting, at least for the younger patients, that depression is not simply a reaction to illness. This study also suggests that further research should perhaps investigate early-onset and late-onset Parkinson's disease as separate illnesses with different clinical courses.

When depression is found to precede the clinical motor picture of Parkinson's disease, could this depression be the first symptom of the disease? For example, could mild degeneration of catecholamine systems produce depression and more advanced degeneration result in the motor symptoms? Alternatively, because depression is a common illness in the general population, could preexisting depression, which is presumed to be related somehow to changes in neurotransmitter functioning, make a patient more vulnerable to, or allow the earlier expression of, Parkinson's disease? This literature was comprehensively reviewed by Todes and Lees (1985), who noted that these issues remained unresolved.

A more recent study by Hubble and colleagues (1993) reported depression is the third strongest predictor of Parkinson's disease, after pesticide exposure and family history of neurological disease.

Epilepsy

Numerous studies attest to the high incidence of psychiatric problems in epilepsy. Initial studies did not use standardized screening instruments or modern diagnostic categories, but most were consistent in reporting a high incidence of problems confirmed by more modern studies. Among the first American studies was that of Gibbs and colleagues (1948), who reported an increased incidence of hysteria, psychopathic personality, or schizoid psychosis in patients with a psychomotor interictal pattern on electroencephalogram. Pond and Bidwell (1959) reported that 38% of a series of epileptic outpatients had some form of psychiatric illness. Rutter and colleagues (1979) surveyed in detail the entire population of the Isle of Wight and found a 58% incidence of psychiatric problems in 8- to 10-year-old epileptic children. Currie and colleagues (1971) screened 666 patients with complex partial seizures and reported that almost half of this population experienced psychiatric problems.

These initial studies and others were sharply challenged by Stevens (1966), who noted that many of these studies drew on psychiatric clinic populations, lacked appropriate control subjects, and were unstandardized, invalidating the conclusion. She observed that as of 1966, only three studies had compared the incidence of psychiatric disability in psychomotor and nonpsychomotor seizure patients who were matched for age and unselected by derivation from a psychiatric source. These were Vislie and Henrikson (1958) from Oslo, Norway; Guerrant (1962) from San Francisco, California; and Jul-Jensen (1964) from Scandinavia. None of these found a difference in psychiatric morbidity between psychomotor and other forms of epilepsy. These studies, however, did show a high incidence of psychiatric problems for the entire group. Even Stevens herself, who stringently defined psychiatric disturbance as a history of a prior psychiatric hospitalization, found that 28 of 100 randomly selected epileptic patients qualified. Pritchard and colleagues (1980) performed a similar study of a group of 56 carefully defined patients with partial seizures between the ages of 15 and 30 years. Psychiatric disturbance—defined as a history of admission to a psychiatric hospital, suicide attempt, referral to psychiatry, or behavioral disturbance—was found in 37%.

Depression is the most commonly reported psychiatric complication of epilepsy. Epileptic patients have a suicide rate at least five times that of the general population (Barraclough 1981; Matthews and Barbas 1981). Mendez and colleagues (1986) reported that 78% of psychiatric hospitalizations of epileptic patients were for some form of affective disorder. They anecdotally stated that most patients denied feeling a loss of control, social stigmatization, and so on, and that for most, epilepsy was an accepted lifelong problem that did not appear to contribute to their depression.

Noting methodological shortcomings of prior studies, Kogeorgas and colleagues (1982) studied the incidence of psychiatric morbidity in a series of 66 patients drawn from an outpatient clinic for epilepsy. Patients who had the onset of a psychiatric disorder prior to the onset of epilepsy were excluded. (Given the difficulty of determining the onset of partial seizures, this probably lowered the true incidence.) Patients were matched with a control group of neurological patients without epilepsy. All patients were given the General Health Questionnaire and Crown-

Crisp Experiential Index. Sufficient General Health Questionnaire scores were found in 45% of the epileptic patients, 28% of the neurological control subjects, and 21% of a previously derived community sample to indicate "probable psychiatric cases." Depression, anxiety, and hysteria were the most commonly reported characteristics.

An elegant and exhaustive review of possible organic contributions to depressive illness in epilepsy has been published by Robertson (1989). She noted that although there is substantial evidence that depression is common in persons with epilepsy, there is as yet no consensus on characteristics or causes of this depression. Although multiple causes have been implicated—including the structural and neurotransmitter alterations of epilepsy, the role of anticonvulsants, and social stigmatization—no studies have addressed in a systematic way whether depression is more common in epileptic patients than in other neurological patients.

Patient compliance is far more important in epilepsy than in most other illnesses. A patient with aphasia will be aphasic no matter what he or she does. Whether a patient will have seizures, however, is to a large extent dependent on the patient's compliance with a usually complex medical regimen involving multiple daily doses, frequent office visits, and medical tests. Therefore, psychological feelings of denial or depression that affect compliance can have a large impact on the course of the disease. Because individual psychodynamics are linked to family dynamics, family pathology also adversely affects the course of epilepsy. Dodrill (1983), discussing the psychological problems of epilepsy, commented that there is no standard definition of a psychosocial problem and that there is no universal agreement as to which problems exist. In an effort to systematize investigation in this area, Dodrill and colleagues (Dodrill 1983; Dodrill et al. 1980) developed a framework to classify in objective and comprehensive terms the problems encountered in epilepsy. They introduced the Washington Psychological Seizure Inventory, which identifies eight areas of concern: family background, emotional adjustment, interpersonal adjustment, vocational adjustment, financial status, adjustment to seizures, medical care, and overall psychosocial functioning.

Levin and colleagues (1988) comprehensively reviewed the available literature on psychological problems in epilepsy, using the framework developed by Dodrill and colleagues (Dodrill 1983; Dodrill et al. 1980).

They noted the major methodological limitations of most studies, including sample size, lack of control subjects, inadequate or nonexistent measures of behavior, and unaddressed confounding variables (e.g., diagnostic clarity, medication, and intelligence). Although the bulk of the literature indicated that psychosocial problems exist, Levin and colleagues found that the association between specific emotional adjustment problems and epilepsy was not conclusive and was often contradictory. This suggests that although psychosocial problems in epilepsy are an important subject for future research, it is premature to include such problems in a nosological classification system such as the DSM.

Discussion

There is abundant evidence that psychiatric illness is commonly associated with a broad range of neurological disorders. This understanding evolved as psychiatry itself developed. Initial reports of psychological factors in neurological disease were anecdotal, although more recent efforts have classified and better delineated the nature of the psychiatric disturbance in terms of (constantly changing) diagnostic categories. Moreover, there has been a clear shift from viewing mental processes as somehow independent of brain functioning to viewing psychiatric symptoms in terms of neurophysiology. A major obstacle, as far as the focal instance of depression is concerned, has been the absence of a reliable and objective biological marker. This has some parallel in the history of science for many other illnesses. Earlier in this century, for example, MS could not be separated antemortem from general paresis and other disorders because of the absence of reliable and objective diagnostic markers. Our understanding of MS did progress despite this, although progress was slow and hampered by many false leads. A major advance in those days was the introduction of the Schumacher Criteria for MS (Schumacher et al. 1965), a checklist of symptoms and signs that investigators could use to define MS for further research, a checklist not at all unlike those found in the DSM.

Because, however, all the central nervous system illnesses discussed here entail a diseased brain by definition, the distinctions among organic mood disorders, adjustment disorders, major depression, and so forth in this context become very blurred and have been avoided here. The bulk of the evidence suggests that we do not yet have sufficient information to make these distinctions. For example, when depression complicates Parkinson's disease (or any other illnesses), does the depression precipitate the disease by lowering the reserve of neurotransmitters? Or is the depression the first sign of Parkinson's disease, with the motor complications (such as cogwheeling and tremor) appearing only later as the disease progresses? Because the answer is not known, major depression cannot be confidently separated from organic mood disorder, even when the depressive illness antedates Parkinson's disease by several years. By extension, it becomes problematic to separate any fragment of affect or behavior, or any "psychological characteristic," from the underlying neurological process.

Recommendations

Our understanding of the relationship of psychiatric to neurological disease improves when investigators make clear, explicit, and empiric descriptions of the disorder they are studying. For example, studies have determined that patients may have identical MMSE or HRSD scores and yet be quite different in presentation (Anthony et al. 1982; Beatty and Goodkin 1990; Franklin et al. 1988). Also, as argued cogently by Taylor and Saint-Cyr (1990), overlap between the symptoms of depression and of neurological illness might cause false inflation of the rating scores for depression. Detailed descriptions of objective findings allow results to be carried over when diagnostic standards change, as they have done significantly over the last several decades.

Distinctions should be made, when possible, between temporal associations, which are observed, and causal associations, which are inferred—particularly because the pathophysiology of psychiatric illness is so poorly understood. This very lack of knowledge, however, makes the exploration of psychiatric disease in neurological illness crucial because such exploration promises a better understanding of the basic mechanism of psychiatric illness.

References

American Psychiatric Association: Diagnostic and Statistical Manual of Mental Disorders, 3rd Edition. Washington, DC, American Psychiatric Association, 1980

American Psychiatric Association: Diagnostic and Statistical Manual of Mental Disorders, 3rd Edition, Revised. Washington, DC, American Psychiatric Association, 1987

American Psychiatric Association: Diagnostic and Statistical Manual of Mental Disorders, 4th Edition. Washington, DC, American Psychiatric Association, 1994

Anthony JC, Le Resche L, Niaz V, et al: Limits of the "Mini Mental State" as a screening test for dementia and delirium among hospitalized patients. Psychol Med 12:397–408, 1982

Barraclough B: Suicide and epilepsy, in Epilepsy and Psychiatry. Edited by Reynolds EH, Trimble MR. New York, Churchill Livingstone, 1981, pp 72–76

Barry Jr, Dunteman GH, Webb MW: Personality and motivation in rehabilitation. Journal of Counselling Psychology 15:237–244, 1968

Beatty WW, Goodkin DE: Screening of cognitive impairment in multiple sclerosis: an evaluation of the Mini-Mental State Examination. Arch Neurol 47:297–301, 1990

Benson DF: Psychiatric aspects of aphasia. Br J Psychiatry 123:555–566, 1973

Bolla-Wilson K, Robinson RG, Starkstein SE, et al: Lateralization dementia and depression in stroke patients. Am J Psychiatry 146:627–634, 1989

Boyle EA, Clark CM, Klonoff H, et al: Empirical support for psychological profiles observed in multiple sclerosis. Arch Neurol 48:1150–1154, 1991

Braceland FJ, Giffen ME: The mental changes associated with multiple sclerosis (an interim report). Res Publ Assoc Res Nerv Ment Dis 28:450–455, 1950

Brown LG, Wilson WP: Parkinsonism and depression. South Med J 65:540–545, 1972

Brown S, Davis TK: The mental symptoms of multiple sclerosis. Archives of Neurology and Psychiatry 7:629–634, 1922

Cantello R, Gilli M, Riccio A, et al: Mood changes associated with "end-of-dose deterioration" in Parkinson's disease: a controlled investigation. J Neurol Neurosurg Psychiatry 49:1182–1190, 1986

Celesia GG, Wannamaker WM: Psychiatric disturbances in Parkinson's disease. Diseases of the Nervous System 33:577–583, 1972

Charatan FB, Fish A: The mental and emotional results of strokes. N Y State J Med 78:1403–1405, 1978

Cherington MR: Parkinsonism, L-dopa and mental depression. J Am Geriatr Soc 18:513–516, 1970

Cogswell BE: Self-socialization readjustment of paraplegics in community. Journal of Rehabilitation 34:11–13, 1968

Cottrell SS, Wilson SA: The affective symptomatology of disseminated sclerosis. Journal of Neurology and Psychopathology 7:1–20, 1926

Currie S, Heathfield KW, Henson RA, et al: Clinical courses and prognosis of temporal lobe epilepsy: a survey of 666 patients. Brain 94:173–190, 1971

Dalos NP, Rabins PV, Brooks BR, et al: Disease activity and emotional state in multiple sclerosis. Ann Neurol 13:573–577, 1983

Dodrill CB: Psychosocial characteristics of epileptic patients, in Epilepsy. Edited by Ward AA Jr, Penry JK, Purpura D. New York, Raven, 1983, pp 341–353

Dodrill CB, Batzel LW, Queisser HR, et al: An objective method for the assessment of psychological and social problems among epileptics. Epilepsia 21:123–135, 1980

Foley FW, Traugott U, LaRocca NG, et al: A prospective study of depression and immune dysregulation in multiple sclerosis. Arch Neurol 49:238–244, 1992

Folstein MF, Mailberger R, McHugh PR: Mood disorder as a specific complication of stroke. J Neurol Neurosurg Psychiatry 40:2018–2020, 1977

Franklin GM, Heaton RK, Nelson CM, et al: Correlation of neuropsychological and MRI findings in chronic/progressive multiple sclerosis. Neurology 38:1826–1829, 1988

Geschwind N: The organization of language and the brain. Science 170:940–944, 1970

Gibbs EL, Giffs FA, Fuster B: Psychomotor epilepsy. Archives of Neurology and Psychiatry 60:331–339, 1948

Guerrant JS: Personality in Epilepsy. Springfield, IL, Charles C Thomas, 1962

Homer WG, Hurwitz T, Li DKB, et al: Temporal lobe involvement in multiple sclerosis patients with psychiatric disorders. Arch Neurol 44:187–190, 1987

Hubble JP, Cao T, Hassanein RES, et al: Risk factors for Parkinson's disease. Neurology 43:1693–1697, 1993

Hyman MD: Social psychological determinants of patients' performance in stroke rehabilitation. Arch Phys Med Rehabil 53:217–226, 1972a

Hyman MD: Sociopsychological obstacles to L-dopa therapy that may limit effectiveness in parkinsonism. J Am Geriatr Soc 20:200–208, 1972b

Joffe RT, Lippert GP, Gray TA, et al: Mood disorder and multiple sclerosis. Arch Neurol 44:376–378, 1987

Jul-Jensen P: Epilepsy: a clinical and social analysis of 1020 adult patients with epileptic seizures. Acta Neurol Scand 40 (suppl 5):1–148, 1964

Kahana E, Leibowitz U, Alter M: Cerebral multiple sclerosis. Neurology 21:1179–1185, 1971

Kogeorgas J, Fonagy P, Scott DF: Psychiatric symptom patterns of chronic epileptics attending a neurological clinic: a controlled investigation. Br J Psychiatry 140:236–243, 1982

Kraepelin E: Psychiatrie ien Lehbuch fur Studierende und Artze (1901), in Clinical Psychiatry. Translated by Diefenorf AR. New York, Macmillan, 1915, pp 335–355

Levin R, Banks S, Berg B: Psychosocial dimensions of epilepsy: a review of the literature. Epilepsia 209:805–816, 1988

Lipsey J, Robinson R, Pearlson G, et al: Nortryptyline treatment of post stroke depression: a double blind study. Lancet 1:297–300, 1985

Lyon-Caen O, Jouvent R, Hauser S, et al: Cognitive function in recent onset demyelinating disease. Arch Neurol 43:1138–1141, 1986

MacGuiffe RA, Janzen FV, Samuelson CO, et al: Self concept and ideal-self in assessing the rehabilitation applicant. Journal of Counselling Psychology 15:157–161, 1969

Marsh GG, Markham CH: Does levodopa alter depression and psychopathology in parkinsonism patients? J Neurol Neurosurg Psychiatry 36:925–935, 1973

Matthews KB: Multiple sclerosis presenting with acute remitting psychiatric symptoms. J Neurol Neurosurg Psychiatry 42:859–863, 1979

Matthews WS, Barbas G: Suicide and epilepsy: a review of the literature. Psychosomatics 22:515–524, 1981

Mayberg HS, Robinson RG, Wond DF, et al: PET imaging of cortical S_2 serotonin receptors after stroke: lateralized changes and relationship to depression. Am J Psychiatry 145:937–943, 1988

Mayeux R, Stern Y, Rosen J, et al: Depression, intellectual impairment, and Parkinson's disease. Neurology 31:645–650, 1981

Mayeux R, Stern Y, Cote L, et al: Altered serotonin metabolism in depressed patients in Parkinson's disease. Neurology 34:642–646, 1984

Mayeux R, Stern Y, Williams JB, et al: Clinical and biochemical features of depression in Parkinson's disease. Am J Psychiatry 143:757–759, 1986

Mayeux R, Stern Y, Sano M, et al: The relationship of serotonin to depression in Parkinson's disease. Mov Disord 3:237–244, 1988

Mendez MF, Cummings JL, Benson F: Depression in epilepsy. Arch Neurol 43:766–770, 1986

Mindham RH: Psychiatric symptoms in parkinsonism. J Neurol Neurosurg Psychiatry 33:181–191, 1970

Pond DA, Bidwell BH: A survey of epilepsy in 14 general practices, II: social and psychological aspects. Epilepsia 60:285–299, 1959

Prichard JS, Schwab RS, Tillman WA: The effects of stress and the results of medication in different personalities with Parkinson's disease. Psychosom Med 13:106–111, 1951

Pritchard PP, Lombroso CT, McIntyre M: Psychological complications of temporal lobe epilepsy. Neurology 30:227–232, 1980

Reding R: Antidepressants after stroke. Arch Neurol 43:762–765, 1986

Riklan M, Weiner H, Diller L: Somato-psychologic studies in Parkinson's disease, I: an investigation into the relationship of certain disease factors to psychological functions. J Nerv Ment Dis 129:263–272, 1959

Robertson NM: The organic contribution to depressive illness in patients with epilepsy. Journal of Epilepsy 2:189–230, 1989

Robins AH: Depression in patients with parkinsonism. Br J Psychiatry 128:141–145, 1976

Robinson RG, Price TR: Post-stroke depressive disorders: a follow-up study of 103 patients. Stroke 13:635–641, 1982

Robinson RG, Starkstein SE: Current research in affective disorders following stroke. Journal of Neuropsychiatry and Clinical Neurosciences 2:1–14, 1990

Robinson RG, Star LB, Kubos KL, et al: A two year longitudinal study of post-stroke mood disorders: findings during the initial evaluation. Stroke 14:736–741, 1983

Robinson RG, Star LB, Price TR, et al: A two year longitudinal study of mood disorders following stroke, prevalence and duration at 6 months follow-up. Br J Psychiatry 144:256–262, 1984

Robinson RG, Bolla-Wilson K, Kaplan E, et al: Depression influences intellectual impairment in stroke patients. Br J Psychiatry 148:541–547, 1986

Rutter M, Graham PJ, Yule W (eds): The prevalence of psychiatric disorder in neuro-epileptic children, in A Neuropsychiatric Study in Childhood. London, Heinman Medical Book, 1979, pp 175–185

Santamaria J, Tolosa E, Valles A: Parkinson's disease with depression: a possible subgroup of idiopathic parkinsonism. Neurology 36:1130–1133, 1986

Schiffer RB: The spectrum of depression in multiple sclerosis. Arch Neurol 44:596–599, 1987

Schiffer RB, Caine ED, Bamford KA, et al: Depressive episodes in patients with multiple sclerosis. Am J Psychiatry 140:1498–1500, 1983

Schiffer RB, Wineman M, Weitkamp LR: Association between bipolar affective disorder and multiple sclerosis. Am J Psychiatry 143:94–95, 1986

Schiffer RB, Kurlan R, Rubin A, et al: Evidence for a typical depression in Parkinson's disease. Am J Psychiatry 145:1020–1022, 1988

Schumacher GA, Beebe G, Kibler RF, et al: Problems of experimental trials of therapy in multiple sclerosis. Ann N Y Acad Sci 122:552–568, 1965

Singer E: Sociological factors influencing response to levodopa therapy for Parkinson's disease. Arch Phys Med Rehabil 57:328–334, 1976

Slater SB, Sussman MB, Stroud MW: Participation in household activities as prognostic factor for rehabilitation. Arch Phys Med Rehabil 51:605–610, 1970

Spitzer RL, Endicott J, Robins E: Research Diagnostic Criteria: rationale and reliability. Arch Gen Psychiatry 35:773–782, 1978

Starkstein SE, Berthier ML, Bolduc PL, et al: Depression in patients with early versus late onset of Parkinson's disease. Neurology 39:1441–1445, 1989

Stevens JR: Psychiatric implications of psychomotor epilepsy. Arch Gen Psychiatry 14:461–471, 1966

Surridge D: An investigation into some psychiatric aspects of multiple sclerosis. Br J Psychiatry 115:749–764, 1969

Taylor AE, Saint-Cyr JA: Depression in Parkinson's disease: reconciling physiological and psychological perspectives. Journal of Neuropsychiatry and Clinical Neurosciences 2:92–98, 1990

Todes CH, Lees AJ: The premorbid personality of patients with Parkinson's disease. J Neurol Neurosurg Psychiatry 48:97–100, 1985

Vislie H, Henrikson GF: Psychic disturbance in epileptics, in Lectures on Epilepsy. Edited by Lorentz de Haas A. Amsterdam, Elsevier, 1958, pp 29–90

Warburton JW: Depressive symptoms in parkinsonism patients referred for thalamotomy. J Neurol Neurosurg Psychiatry 30:368–370, 1967

Wechsler IS: Statistics of multiple sclerosis including a study of the infantile, congenital, familial and hereditary forms and the mental and psychic symptoms. Archives of Neurology and Psychiatry 8:59–75, 1921

Whitlock FA, Siskind MM: Depression as a major symptom of multiple sclerosis. J Neurol Neurosurg Psychiatry 43:861–865, 1980

Young AC, Saunders J, Ponsford JR: Mental change as an early feature of multiple sclerosis. J Neurol Neurosurg Psychiatry 39:1008–1013, 1976

CHAPTER 5

Cancer Onset and Progression

JAMES L. LEVENSON, M.D.

CLAUDIA BEMIS, M.D.

Many professionals and laypersons believe that psychological factors play a major role in cancer onset and progression. The media have promoted popular ideas of overcoming cancer through "mind over body," and there are self-help books and retreat centers where patients can learn imagery and relaxation techniques to fight their cancer. Guided imagery (visualizing white cells attacking cancer cells), cognitive restructuring (thinking positive thoughts), and assertiveness training have all been promoted alongside traditional health care for the cancer patient to "combat" disease.

Enthusiasm for these optimistic theories and practices should be tempered by the recognition that scientific evidence supporting a relationship between psychological factors and cancer lags far behind. In part, this may be due to the complexities involved in studying cancer, for a host of factors may contribute to onset and progression. In this chapter we review the scientific evidence pertaining to the major psychological factors that have been studied. Many existing reports are limited by flawed research design and analysis, which is also discussed.

From a historical perspective, the 1950s witnessed a surge of interest in psychosomatic medicine and in research linking psychological, social, and environmental factors to disease onset and progression. A major finding was the association between smoking and lung cancer. In the following decade, personality traits, conflicts, and affects were examined as possible contributors to the onset and promotion of many diseases, including cancer. Exposures to certain environmental and occupational toxins were also linked to several cancers. The 1960s likewise witnessed the growth of experiments using animals in the hope of better understanding the effects of psychological and behavioral factors on cancer while controlling confounding variables. Extrapolating conclusions from these studies that can apply to humans remains problematic and is discussed later. The 1970s saw rapid advances in immunology and neurochemistry, and psychiatry became more involved with the biological basis of mental disorders. Intriguing associations between certain affective states and the neuroendocrine system were demonstrated. Further research in the 1980s in psychoneuroimmunology explored relationships between immunological response and psychosocial variables as well as the implications for cancer vulnerability and progression (Holland 1989).

In this chapter, we look at two hypotheses, along with the positive and negative studies associated with them: 1) cancer onset and progression are affected by psychosocial variables; and 2) psychological factors affect the immune system, which in turn can contribute to cancer onset and progression. Psychosocial variables examined here include affective states, coping/defensive styles and personality traits, interpersonal variables, and stressful life events. The impact of psychosocial interventions on cancer outcome and animal models are also discussed.

Although extensive research in psychooncology has appeared over the decades, much of it is methodologically flawed. Flaws have included use of small and biased samples, heterogeneous samples that mixed patients with very different cancer types or at different stages, limited or no statistical analysis, poor controls, and retrospective subject bias. Several studies that seemed to show significant effects were inconclusive because of nonequivalence in groups at baseline either in disease severity or in therapy received (many studies did not even monitor this possibility). Some studies failed to attend to important potential confounding factors such as smoking or diet. A number of studies measured too many psychological variables and then overemphasized the few "discovered" positive associations in published results. Failure to standardize measures of initial psychological factors and measures of medical outcome has also been frequent.

Methods

Extensive reviews of this topic were already available (Fox 1983; Holland 1989; Spiegel and Sands 1993) and were supplemented with *Index*

Medicus and MedLine searches through 1989. Studies were not included if they were judged seriously flawed methodologically (as noted above). Very few studies met the full set of criteria. Given the limitations of reviewing an extremely small number of studies, we also included other studies that, based on our qualitative judgment, had methodological strengths that outweighed their flaws.

Psychosocial Variables

Affective States

The linking of affective states, particularly depression, with the onset of cancer has been an active area of study. One large epidemiologic study of 2,020 male employees of Western Electric reported that depressive symptoms on the Minnesota Multiphasic Personality Inventory (MMPI) were associated with twice as high a risk of death from cancer 17 years later and with a higher-than-normal incidence of cancer for the first 10 years (Shekelle et al. 1981). This finding persisted at 20-year follow-up (Persky et al. 1987). The Western Electric study has been cited for many years as supporting the association between depressive symptoms and increased cancer risk. On critically reexamining these data, however, Bieliauskas and Garron (1982) found that the depression scores that were reported to be "high" were not in the pathological range.

More recent epidemiologic studies have demonstrated negative findings. In a prospective cohort study of 9,832 women over a period of 10–14 years follow-up, Hahn and Petitti (1988) failed to find an association between MMPI depression scores and breast cancer in women who were initially cancer free. Severe depression reflected by MMPI depression scores of ≥70 also showed no correlation. Kaplan and Reynolds (1988) studied 688 healthy subjects prospectively over 17 years for the development of cancer. Subjects completed an 18-item self-rating depression index. No association was found between the development of cancer and depression. Weissman and colleagues (1986) followed 515 randomly selected subjects over 6 years and found that depressive symptoms (on the Self-Assessment Depression Scale) did not predict subsequent mortality. Dattore and colleagues (1980) found significantly *lower* MMPI depression scores in men who subsequently developed any type of cancer. A study by Zonderman and colleagues (1989) with a 10-year follow-up from the National Health and Nutrition Examination Survey found no significant depressive symptoms (using the Cheerful versus Depressed subscale from the General Well-Being Schedule and the Center for Epidemiologic Studies Depression Scale) that could be seen as predictors of cancer morbidity or mortality.

In general, most studies examining depressive states are flawed by their lack of specification. Most investigators have not differentiated among various depressive disorders and have not examined depressions from the perspective of past history, duration, chronicity, or treatment pursued. Whether or not differences in depressive states might influence cancer outcome (e.g., characterologic depressions versus melancholic depressions) remains unknown. Many reports have regarded feelings of hopelessness and helplessness as equivalent to the presence of depression. Additionally, it is problematic to compare studies that use different instruments to measure the presence of depression. Instruments vary in whether they are designed to measure depressive states, traits, or clinical depression, which further confounds cross-comparison of studies. Another problem is that studies often do not control for other relevant psychosocial variables. For example, depression precipitated by loss of a significant other may be confounded by changes in coping/defensive styles or changes in habits such as excessive alcohol intake, poor diet, or increased social isolation. A more complete review of depression and cancer can be found elsewhere (Bieliauskas and Garron 1982).

Few studies have systematically examined the prevalence of psychiatric disorders among cancer patients, and, of these, many have been limited by biased samples and instruments that measure symptoms rather than diagnoses. In contrast, Derogatis and colleagues (1983) assessed 215 cancer patients using explicit DSM-III (American Psychiatric Association 1980) diagnostic criteria. The results indicated that 47% of the patients received a DSM-III diagnosis, including 44% with an Axis I disorder and 12% with a personality disorder. Approximately 68% of the psychiatric diagnoses consisted of adjustment disorders, whereas 13% (6% of the entire sample) represented major affective disorders (i.e., major depression and/or dysthymic disorder). This prevalence rate is close to the 6-month prevalence rate for major affective disorders in the general population found in the Epidemiologic Catchment Area study (Myers et al. 1984).

Besides epidemiologic studies, other research has focused on the impact of affective states on outcome in cancer patients. Studies examining the effect of depression on cancer outcome in clinical samples most often have focused on breast cancer. Much of the data have been retrospective and can be criticized not only for lack of controls, but also for the bias that exists when patients who know their diagnosis are queried about lifestyle and affective states. Another problem with most studies of depression and cancer has been that few studies have measured lifetime prevalence of depression. In a report by Greer and colleagues (1979), breast cancer patients who demonstrated a "fighting spirit" or who used denial had a higher survival rate than those with stoic acceptance or expressed hopelessness and helplessness. This study has been criticized, however, for not controlling for stage of disease. Other clinical studies also have not found a relationship between depression and cancer outcome (Cassileth et al. 1985; Jamison et al. 1987).

Anecdotal reports have long noted that depression is sometimes the presenting symptom of pancreatic cancer, occurring well before symptoms of the tumor begin (Fras et al. 1968; Pomara and Gershon 1984; Savage and Noble 1954; Yaskin 1931). Whether this represents a prodrome or a form of paraneoplastic syndrome remains controversial. Studies have confirmed that depression occurs with greater frequency and severity in pancreatic cancer than in other gastrointestinal cancers, but the underlying mechanism remains obscure (Shakin and Holland 1988).

Bereavement has been recognized as a significant stressor and often has been assumed to be a risk factor in cancer onset and progression. An early retrospective study showed that the onset of hematologic malignancy appeared to be preceded by significant losses in children and young adults (Greene et al. 1956). Other studies have not shown bereavement to be a factor in the development or progression of cancer (Greer et al. 1979; Helsing and Szklo 1981; Klerman and Clayton 1984). Epidemiologic studies are lacking in this area. Bereavement is associated with a significant increase in mortality in the first year in men younger than 75 years of age. However, an examination of the causes of death has shown that accidents, cardiovascular disease, some infectious diseases, and cirrhosis have contributed to the increase, whereas cancer has not. In addition, bereaved women do not show an increase in mortality due to cancer. Thus, bereavement has not been shown to be a factor in cancer onset and progression.

New interest in bereavement has been triggered by studies showing depressed immune function during acute grief (Bartrop et al. 1977; Schleifer et al. 1983). However, depressed levels of immune function were not pathologically low in these studies. Irwin and colleagues (1987) examined natural killer (NK) cell activity and T cell subpopulations in three groups of women: those experiencing bereavement, those anticipating their husband's death from lung cancer, and a control group. NK cell activity was significantly lower in both groups compared with control subjects, with the most depressed subjects demonstrating the most reduced NK activity and changes in the ratio of T helper to T suppressor cells. These studies provide intriguing data, but it is premature to draw conclusions about whether depressed immune function can influence cancer onset or progression.

Coping/Defensive Style and Personality Traits

A large body of literature has described the cancer patient's degree of emotional expressiveness and its purported effect on prognosis. Descriptive case reports began appearing in the 1950s, noting shorter survival in patients with depressed, resigning characteristics compared with patients who were able to express more negative emotions, such as anger. However, many studies were flawed by a failure to control for staging and other confounding variables. In a 30-year follow-up study of 972 physicians, it was reported that "loners" were much more likely to develop cancer than the group characterized by "acting-out" and emotional expression, although potential confounding variables were not examined (Shaffer et al. 1987). Temoshok and Heller (1981) conceptualized "expressive" versus "repressive" variables in terms of a Type C behavior pattern. The Type C individual was described as a cooperative, unassertive patient who suppresses negative emotions, particularly anger, and who accepts or complies with external authorities. The Type C behavior pattern contrasts with Type A, which has been studied as a factor in the development of coronary artery disease. The relationship between Type C and melanoma tumor thickness and invasion was investigated. Tumor thickness and measures of Type C personality correlated, particularly in subjects under the age of 55 years (Temoshok et al. 1985). Kneier and Temoshok (1984) also found that melanoma patients were more "repressed" on self-report measures of repressiveness than were both cardiovascular patients and disease-free control subjects. The Melbourne Colorectal Cancer Study found that cancer patients are more likely to have certain personality traits (very similar to the Type C pattern) than control subjects (Kune et al. 1991a). A study by Greer and colleagues (1979) showed that breast cancer patients who used denial or who possessed a "fighting spirit" survived longer than those patients who demonstrated hopelessness and helplessness, although the stage of disease was not controlled.

Negative studies have also appeared (e.g., Cassileth et al. 1985), showing that none of the multiple psychosocial factors thought to be predictive of health (including hopelessness/helplessness) predicted cancer survival (see also Holland 1989; Jamison et al. 1987). The study by Cassileth and colleagues has been criticized because it used melanoma patients with primarily advanced disease, at which point the role of psychological factors would be likely to have less of an influence. Epidemiologic studies have not supported a relationship between emotional repression and cancer incidence or mortality (Persky et al. 1987; Ragland et al. 1987; Shekelle et al. 1981).

Interpersonal Variables

Relatively less research has examined the effects of interpersonal variables on cancer. One prospective study of former medical students reported that lack of closeness with their parents and less satisfactory relationships were associated with later development of cancer (Graves et al. 1991). A prospective study of breast cancer patients found a number of positive relationship variables predictive of increased survival (Waxler-Morrison et al. 1991). Social relations and social support and their effects on cancer patients (as with other diseases) are complex phenomena and may vary with cancer site and extent of disease (Ell et al. 1992).

Stressful Life Events

Interest in this area has been particularly stimulated by animal studies that have shown that stress in animals can hasten the onset of viral-induced cancer in susceptible strains. Other studies have shown that stress can enhance the carcinogenic potential of several known mutagens in animal subjects. Animal studies demonstrating negative findings also exist and have shown that under certain conditions stress can reduce susceptibility or delay the "take" of implanted tumors. Fox (1983) extensively critiqued both the positive and negative findings in animal studies.

A number of human studies have shown an increased incidence of stressful life events preceding the onset of cervical, pancreatic, gastric, and lung cancers (Ernster et al. 1979; Fras et al. 1967; Horne and Picard 1979; Leherer 1980; Schmale and Iker 1965) and more recently in colorectal cancer (Kune et al. 1991b) and breast cancer (Geyer 1991). One study explicitly linked stress to cancer progression, although the findings were equivocally age dependent (Funch and Marshall 1983). Ramirez and colleagues (1989) demonstrated an association between stressful life events and the first recurrence of operable breast cancer. The limitations of this study included a small number of subjects ($N = 50$) and a retrospective design. Many other studies have failed to find any association between preceding stressful life events and cancer onset (Finn et al. 1974; Graham et al. 1971; Greer and Morris 1975; Grissom et al. 1975; Snell and Graham 1971). Keehn and colleagues (1974) found no excess in cancer during a 24-year follow-up of World War II veterans who were discharged with a diagnosis of (war-related) psychoneurosis. In addition, no increase in cancer rate was demonstrated in prisoners of war from three wars (Keehn 1980). In 1983, on the basis of the sum of human and animal studies, Fox concluded that if stressful events or other psychological factors do have an effect on cancer incidence, it is small. This conclusion would be appropriate today.

Psychosocial Intervention and Cancer Outcome

Several studies have shown improvement in the quality of life in cancer patients receiving group therapy, including improved mood and vigor, decreased pain, and better adjustment (Fawzy et al. 1990a; Grossarth-Maticek et al. 1984; Spiegel et al. 1989). However, not until more recently have well-controlled studies documented increased survival time in cancer patients receiving psychotherapy.

Grossarth-Maticek and colleagues (1984) studied women with metastatic breast cancer, including one group receiving chemotherapy and a group who had declined it. Within each of these two groups, women were randomly assigned to receive or not to receive psychotherapy. Survival was longer in patients who received psychotherapy alone or chemotherapy alone compared with patients who received no treatment; survival was longest in those who received both psychotherapy and chemotherapy, with apparent synergistic effects.

Spiegel and colleagues (Spiegel and Bloom 1983; Spiegel et al. 1981, 1989) randomly assigned metastatic breast cancer patients to 1 year of psychosocial treatment consisting of weekly supportive group therapy with training in self-hypnosis for pain control. The control group had routine oncologic care. At 1 year, the psychotherapy treatment group had less mood disturbance and fewer phobic responses (Spiegel et al. 1981), and they complained of half as much pain (Spiegel and Bloom 1983). At 10-year follow-up the mean survival time had been 34.8 months for the group randomized to psychotherapy as opposed to 18.9 months for the control group. The authors had expected to, and did, find a beneficial effect of treatment on mood and vigor but had not expected that psychosocial treatment would affect survival. Greater longevity in their sample was associated with less mood disturbance and higher ratings on vigor (Spiegel et al. 1989). Spiegel and colleagues speculated on how the benefits of group psychotherapy for cancer patients can be explained. They hypothesized that patients received social support through the group, which provided an atmosphere in which they could express their feelings and feel accepted. The group may also have allowed patients to problem solve more effectively and thereby to achieve better compliance with their medical programs. Better pain control and control of anxiety and depression may also have contributed to better self-care habits such as diet and exercise.

Fawzy and colleagues (1990a) evaluated the immediate and prolonged effects of a 6-week structured psychiatric group intervention for postsurgical patients with malignant melanoma. Patients who received the intervention had higher vigor than control subjects at 6 weeks and less depression, fatigue, and total mood disturbance at a 6-month follow-up. Experimental subjects demonstrated more active coping than control subjects both at the conclusion of the intervention and at follow-up. This study was the first to examine group psychiatric intervention in patients with early-stage cancer and good prognosis. At follow-up 6 years later, the intervention group showed a lower rate of death (3 of 34) and a trend toward less recurrence (7 of 34), compared with the control patients (10 of 34 and 13 of 34, respectively) (Fawzy et al. 1993).

Psychological Factors and the Immune System

Behavioral immunology is the study of the interaction between psychosocial variables and the immune system. Do psychosocial variables act via the immune system to influence cancer onset and progression? Two separate lines of research shed light on such a postulated relationship, corresponding to two linked hypothesis: 1) psychosocial variables influence the immune system, and 2) the immune system influences cancer onset and progression.

Bereavement as a psychological response to the loss of a relationship has been shown in many studies to alter aspects of immune function. An extensive review of this literature is available elsewhere (Holland 1989). Kiecolt-Glaser and colleagues (Kiecolt-Glaser et al. 1984, 1986) demonstrated that NK cell activity varies with stress and lack of social support. Levy and colleagues (1990b) found an association between perceived level of social support and NK cell activity in 120 stage I and stage II breast cancer patients.

The complex relationships among the various components of the immune system as well as the immune components that may serve as markers of clinical significance in cancer development and outcome are unknown. NK cells are a subclass of lymphocytes, believed to be derived from T cell lines, which are thought to serve in malignant cell surveillance by recognizing and destroying mutant cells that may have precancerous programs.

Studies that have demonstrated altered immune function associated with psychosocial factors have *not* been able to demonstrate a further connection to cancer onset and progression. Confounding variables, such as genetic makeup, that may influence immune efficiency and susceptibility to stresses (both psychological and physiologic) have not been accounted for in human studies demonstrating psychosocial influences on immune function.

The hypothesis that immune function is involved in cancer surveillance has been demonstrated in animal studies showing that immunosuppressed rodents develop tumors not specific to site. Humans who are immunosuppressed can also develop tumors at multiple sites. However, it is still too early to discuss an integrative model for cancer onset and progression that acts via the immune system under the influence of psychosocial variables.

Research has illuminated psychosocial and immune interactions and outcome in individuals who already have cancer. Levy and colleagues (Levy et al. 1985, 1987) examined NK cell activity and three distress indicators in women with breast cancer at the time of mastectomy and 3 months after. They found that adjustment level, lack of social support, fatigue, and depressive symptoms accounted for 30% of the NK cell variance seen at 3 months. In this group, more metastatic nodes were also associated with depressive features and decreased NK cell activity. Subsequent work by this group has suggested that complex relationships exist between psychosocial factors (especially social support), NK cell activity, receptor status, and breast cancer recurrence (Levy et al. 1990a, 1991). The sustained beneficial psychological outcomes with psychiatric group intervention in postsurgical patients with malignant melanoma reported by Fawzy and colleagues (1990a) have been described above. They also found that experimental subjects had significant increases in particular NK cell types and increased NK cytotoxic activity at 6-month follow-up (Fawzy et al. 1990b).

Animal Models

Many experiments examining psychological factors affecting cancer have used animal models, particularly in studying the relationship between stress and cancer onset and progression. Extrapolation of these results to humans can be dangerously misleading. Key differences between cancer in experimental animals and cancer in humans should be noted. Rodent strains that are highly inbred may be more susceptible to developing cancers; and many spontaneous cancers in animals are viral, contrasting with only 2%–3% of known cancers that are viral in humans. Potentially confounding variables include 1) external factors such as the quality, quantity, and time course of the stressor; 2) coexisting factors such as diet, parity, and housing of animals; and 3) factors of the internal milieu preexisting viral invasion, genetic susceptibility, and immunocompetence of the organism. Heavy doses of carcinogens are typically used in animal experiments, yielding tumors with strong antigens that may facilitate detection by the immune system. By contrast, in "natural" human cancer, most carcinogens are low-dose and long-acting, presumably yielding weaker antigens that might escape immune surveillance (Spiegel and Bloom 1983).

The human paradigm for cancer cell surveillance is less well known, but, in addition to the immune system, DNA repair may contribute additional protection. Animal studies will continue to help us understand many of the complex variables involved with cancer onset and progression only if we are careful not to draw premature conclusions from them about human cancers. As noted earlier, depending on the animal model and experimental paradigm chosen, stress has been shown to increase and to decrease cancer development and progression.

Discussion

In summary, a number of studies have lent some support to the relationship between a variety of psychological factors and the onset, exacerbation, or outcome of neoplastic disease. At present, no clear associations or causal relationships have been proven, both because of methodological limitations in the positive studies and because of other studies of comparable methodology that have failed to find such relationships.

Compared with other known risk factors, psychosocial factors may by themselves make a small contribution to cancer onset. However, more recent, methodologically sounder studies have suggested that cancer progression, rather than onset, may be more influenced by psychosocial factors. Clearly, better systematically designed research is needed to elucidate further the impact of psychological factors on cancer. Future studies will need to control for staging, the type of cancer and treatment, and confounding variables such as smoking and other risk-associated behaviors. They also will need to include well-matched control subjects.

The gap that currently exists between our scientific knowledge base and popular beliefs about cancer onset and progression can be problematic for individuals with cancer and their health care providers. How can cancer patients distinguish between the popular ideas based on fact and those founded on myth? Are cancer patients responsible for their disease because they did not have the "right attitude" or personality characteristics that would have enhanced their disease resistance? Does seeking a cure for cancer in "love and miracles" complement or undermine standard cancer care? There are some beliefs that exist about cancer onset and progression that may not be empirically supported but that nevertheless can contribute to a patient's sense of well-being and control, whereas others may have an adverse impact. Although psychosocial interventions are more likely to contribute to quality than to quantity of life in cancer patients, their proper scope of application remains to be worked out.

Finally, scarce resource allocation needs to be directed at psychosocial interventions that have empirical support. With better systematic studies, we should have a clearer understanding of where resources should be directed in the future.

References

American Psychiatric Association: Diagnostic and Statistical Manual of Mental Disorders, 3rd Edition. Washington, DC, American Psychiatric Association, 1980

Bartrop R, Lazarus L, Luckhurst E, et al: Depressed lymphocyte function after bereavement. Lancet 1:834–836, 1977

Bieliauskas LA, Garron DC: Psychological depression and cancer. Gen Hosp Psychiatry 4:187–195, 1982

Cassileth BR, Lusk EJ, Miller DS, et al: Psychological correlates of survival in advanced malignant disease? N Engl J Med 312:1551–1555, 1985

Dattore PG, Shontz FC, Coyne L: Premorbid personality differentiation of cancer and noncancer groups: a test of the hypothesis of cancer proneness. J Consult Clin Psychol 48:388–394, 1980

Derogatis LR, Morrow GR, Fetting J, et al: The prevalence of psychiatric disorders among cancer patients. JAMA 249:751–757, 1983

Ell K, Mishimoto R, Mediansky L, et al: Social relations, social support and survival among patients with cancer. J Psychosom Res 36:531–541, 1992

Ernster VL, Sucks ST, Selvin S, et al: Cancer incidence by marital status: US Third National Cancer Survey. J Natl Cancer Inst 63:567–585, 1979

Fawzy FI, Cousins N, Fawzy WW, et al: A structured psychiatric intervention for cancer patients, I: changes over time in methods of coping and affective disturbance. Arch Gen Psychiatry 47:720–725, 1990a

Fawzy FI, Kemeny ME, Fawzy W, et al: A structured psychiatric intervention for cancer patients, II: changes over time in immunologic measures. Arch Gen Psychiatry 47:729–735, 1990b

Fawzy FI, Fawzy NW, Hyun CS, et al: Malignant melanoma: effects of an early structured psychiatric intervention, coping, and affective state on recurrence and survival 6 years later. Arch Gen Psychiatry 50:681–689, 1993

Finn F, Mulcahy R, Hickey W: The psychological profiles of coronary and cancer patients, and of matched controls. Ir J Med Sci 143:176–178, 1974

Fox BH: Current theory of psychogenic effects on cancer incidence and prognosis. Journal of Psychosocial Oncology 1:17–31, 1983

Fras I, Litin EM, Pearson JS: Comparison of psychiatric symptoms in carcinoma of the pancreas with those in some other intra-abdominal neoplasms. Am J Psychiatry 123:1553–1556, 1967

Fras I, Litin EM, Bartholomew LG: Mental symptoms as an aid in the early diagnosis of carcinoma of the pancreas. Gastroenterology 55:191–198, 1968

Funch DP, Marshall J: The role of stress, social support and age in survival from breast cancer. J Psychosom Res 27:77–83, 1983

Geyer S: Life events prior to manifestation of breast cancer: a limited prospective study covering eight years before diagnosis. J Psychosom Res 35:355–363, 1991

Graham S, Snell LM, Graham JB, et al: Social trauma in the epidemiology of cancer of the cervix. Journal of Chronic Disease 24:711–735, 1971

Graves PL, Thomas CB, Mead LA: Familial and psychological predictors of cancer. Cancer Detect Prev 15:59–64, 1991

Greene WA, Young LE, Swisher SN: Psychological factors and reticuloendothelial disease. Psychosom Med 18:284–303, 1956

Greer S, Morris T: Psychological attributes of women who develop breast cancer: a controlled study. J Psychosom Res 19:147–153, 1975

Greer S, Morris T, Pettingale KW: Psychological response to breast cancer: effect on outcome. Lancet 2:785–787, 1979

Grissom J, Weiner B, Weiner E: Psychological correlates of cancer. J Consult Clin Psychol 43:113, 1975

Grossarth-Maticek R, Schmidt P, Veter H, et al: Psychotherapy research in oncology, in Health Care and Human Behavior. Edited by Steptoe A, Mathews A. London, Academic Press, 1984, pp 325–342

Hahn RC, Petitti DB: Minnesota Multiphasic Personality Inventory: rated depression and the incidence of breast cancer. Cancer 61:845–848, 1988

Helsing KJ, Szklo M: Mortality after bereavement. Am J Epidemiol 114:41–52, 1981

Holland JC: Behavioral and psychosocial risk factors in cancer: human studies, in Handbook of Psychooncology. Edited by Holland JC, Rowland JH. New York, Oxford University Press, 1989, pp 705–726

Horne RL, Picard RS: Psychosocial risk factors for lung cancer. Psychosom Med 43:431–438, 1979

Irwin M, Daniels M, Weiner H: Immune and neuroendocrine changes during bereavement. Psychiatr Clin North Am 10:449–465, 1987

Jamison RN, Burish TG, Wallston KA: Psychogenic factors in predicting survival of breast cancer patients. J Clin Oncol 5:768–772, 1987

Kaplan GA, Reynolds P: Depression and cancer mortality and morbidity: prospective evidence from the Alameda County study. J Behav Med 11:1–13, 1988

Keehn RJ: Follow-up studies of World War II and Korean conflict prisoners. Am J Epidemiol 111:194–211, 1980

Keehn RJ, Goldberg LD, Beebe GW: Twenty-four year mortality follow-up of army veterans with disability separations for psychoneurosis in 1944. Psychosom Med 36:27–46, 1974

Kiecolt-Glaser JK, Garner W, Speicher C, et al: Psychosocial modifiers of immune competence in medical students. Psychosom Med 46:7–14, 1984

Kiecolt-Glaser JK, Glaser R, Strain EC, et al: Modulation of cellular immunity in medical students. J Behav Med 9:5–21, 1986

Klerman GL, Clayton P: Epidemiologic perspectives on the health consequences of bereavement, in Bereavement: Reactions, Consequences, and Care. Edited by Osterweis M, Soloman F, Green M. Washington, DC, National Academy Press, 1984

Kneier AW, Temoshok L: Repressive coping reactions in patients with malignant melanoma as compared to cardiovascular patients. J Psychosom Res 28:145–155, 1984

Kune GA, Kune S, Watson LF, et al: Personality as a risk factor in large bowel cancer: data from the Melbourne Colorectal Cancer Study. Psychol Med 21:29–41, 1991a

Kune GA, Kune S, Watson LF, et al: Recent life change and large bowel cancer: data from the Melbourne Colorectal Cancer Study. J Clin Epidemiol 44:57–68, 1991b

Leherer S: Life change and gastric cancer. Psychosom Med 42:499–502, 1980

Levy SM, Herberman R, Maluish A, et al: Prognostic risk assessment in primary breast cancer by behavioral and immunological parameters. Health Psychol 4:99–113, 1985

Levy SM, Herberman RB, Lippman M, et al: Correlation of stress factors with sustained depression of natural killer activity and predicted prognosis in patients with breast cancer. J Clin Oncol 5:348–353, 1987

Levy SM, Herberman RB, Lippman M, et al: Immunological and psychosocial predictors of disease recurrence in patients with early-stage breast cancer. Behav Med 17:67–75, 1991

Levy SM, Herberman RB, Lee J, et al: Estrogen receptor concentration and social factors as predictors of natural killer cell activity in early-stage breast cancer patients: confirmation of a model. Nat Immun Cell Growth Regul 9:313–324, 1990a

Levy SM, Herberman RB, Whiteside T, et al: Perceived social support and tumor estrogen/progesterone receptor status as predictors of natural killer cell activity in breast cancer patients. Psychosom Med 52:73–85, 1990b

Myers JK, Weissman MM, Tischel GL, et al: Six-month prevalence of psychiatric disorders in three communities (1980–1983). Arch Gen Psychiatry 41:959–967, 1984

Persky VW, Kempthorne-Rawson J, Shekelle RP: Personality and risk of cancer: 20-year follow-up of the Western Electric Study. Psychosom Med 49:435–449, 1987

Pomara N, Gershon S: Treatment resistant depression in an elderly patient with pancreatic carcinoma: case report. J Clin Psychiatry 45:439–440, 1984

Ragland DR, Brand RJ, Fox BH: Type A behavior and cancer mortality in the Western Collaborative Group Study (abstract). Psychosom Med 49:209, 1987

Ramirez AJ, Craig TK, Watson JP, et al: Stress and relapse of breast cancer. Br Med J 298:291–293, 1989

Savage C, Noble D: Cancer of the pancreas: two cases simulating psychogenic illness. J Nerv Ment Dis 120:62–65, 1954

Schleifer SJ, Keller SE, Camerino M, et al: Suppression of lymphocyte stimulation following bereavement. JAMA 250:374–377, 1983

Schmale AH, Iker HP: The psychological setting of uterine cervical cancer. Ann N Y Acad Sci 125:807–813, 1965

Shaffer JW, Graves PL, Swank RT, et al: Clustering of personality traits in youth and the subsequent development of cancer among physicians. J Behav Med 10:441–447, 1987

Shakin EJ, Holland J: Depression and pancreatic cancer. Journal of Pain and Symptom Management 3:194–198, 1988

Shekelle RB, Raynor WJ Jr, Ostfeld AM, et al: Psychological depression and 17-year risk of death from cancer. Psychosom Med 43:117–126, 1981

Snell L, Graham S: Social trauma as related to cancer of the breast. Br J Cancer 25:721–734, 1971

Spiegel D, Bloom JR: Group therapy and hypnosis reduce metastatic breast carcinoma pain. Psychosom Med 45:333–339, 1983

Spiegel D, Sands SH: Psychological influences on metastatic disease progression, in Progressive States of Malignant Neoplastic Growth. Edited by Kaiser HE. Dordrecht, The Netherlands, Martinus Nijhoff, 1993

Spiegel D, Bloom JR, Yalom ID: Group support for patients with metastatic cancer: a randomized prospective outcome study. Arch Gen Psychiatry 38:527–533, 1981

Spiegel D, Bloom JR, Kraemer HC, et al: Effects of psychosocial treatment on survival of patients with metastatic breast cancer. Lancet 2:888–891, 1989

Temoshok L, Heller B: Stress and "type C" versus epidemiological risk factors in melanoma. Paper presented at the 89th annual convention of the American Psychological Association, Los Angeles, California, August 25, 1981

Temoshok L, Heller BW, Sageviel RW, et al: The relationship of psychological factors of prognostic indicators in cutaneous malignant melanoma. J Psychosom Res 29:139–153, 1985

Waxler-Morrison N, Hislop TG, Mears B, et al: Effects of social relationships on survival for women with breast cancer: a prospective study. Soc Sci Med 33:177–183, 1991

Weissman MM, Myers JK, Thompson WD, et al: Depressive symptoms as a risk factor for mortality and for major depression, in Life-Span Research on the Prediction of Psychopathology. Edited by Erlenmeyer-Kimling L, Miller NE. Hillsdale, NJ, Lawrence Erlbaum, 1986, pp 251–260

Yaskin JC: Nervous symptoms as earliest manifestations of carcinoma of the pancreas. JAMA 96:1664–1668, 1931

Zonderman AB, Costa PT Jr, McCrae RR: Depression as a risk for cancer morbidity and mortality in a nationally representative sample. JAMA 262:1191–1195, 1989

CHAPTER 6

Gastrointestinal Conditions

DAVID G. FOLKS, M.D.

F. CLEVELAND KINNEY, M.D., PH.D.

The association between psychological factors and the gastrointestinal system has been well established (Epstein et al. 1993). For example, experimentally induced emotional stress has been shown to affect gastrointestinal motility (Clouse 1988). Historically, Alexander (1987) identified emotional factors believed to affect disturbances of appetite and eating, swallowing, digestive functions, and eliminative functions. Moreover, syndrome-specific illnesses—such as irritable bowel syndrome, regional enteritis, ulcerative colitis, dyspepsia, and peptic ulcer disease—have frequently been cited in association with psychological factors.

Psychological factors that significantly affect gastroenterological illnesses may also include nutritional or life-style factors or may be intimately related to the disease process per se; alcohol ingestion and tobacco use clearly foster gastric, liver, and pancreatic disorders (Epstein et al. 1993). Thus, in a typical gastroenterologist's practice as many as 60% of the patients will have complaints that are primarily of psychological origin (Switz 1976). Other psychological areas of concern that are pertinent to cases of dyspepsia, peptic ulcer disease, inflammatory or irritable bowel disease, or other specific gastrointestinal conditions may (or may not) simply be stress related. These conditions are undoubtedly influenced, sometimes significantly, by emotional or psychobiological factors (Drossman et al. 1990; Katon 1984; Van Valkenburg et al. 1984).

This chapter is a distillation of the past decade's literature; we identify the psychological factors that are relevant to the understanding of prevalent gastrointestinal disorders. This chapter also represents part of a concerted effort to improve the nosological approach included in DSM-IV (American Psychiatric Association 1994) and is pertinent to those gastro-enterological conditions in which psychological factors play a significant role.

Methods

The literature was surveyed to identify studies and case reports of psychological factors and gastrointestinal disorders. A computerized search located 348 citations, between 1979 and 1990, deemed appropriate for abstract review; 142 of these articles had either used rigorous research design or presented detailed clinical material. The following is a distillation of this pertinent literature; the majority of these articles specifically considered psychological factors and their association with gastroenterological disturbances. Specific syndromes that were frequently studied included dyspepsia, peptic ulcer disease, irritable bowel syndrome, regional enteritis, and ulcerative colitis as well as other general colonic disturbances. Interestingly, the last decade has yielded only a small body of literature, which is based largely on descriptive or retrospective methods. It is hoped that this review will not only increase our understanding of the implications for future research but will also contribute to a refined nosological approach that will result in the use of improved methods of study for gastroenterology and associated psychiatric factors.

Esophageal Disorders

Dysphagia, the sensation of difficulty in swallowing, is a symptom of several physical disorders recently reviewed by Epstein and colleagues (1993) (Table 6–1). Dysphagia is often an indicator of obstruction, especially when it is progressive and the patient cannot swallow solid foods. If neither solids nor liquids are tolerated, the problem is usually due to motor dysfunction. A barium swallow or esophagogram will serve to diagnose the nature of the mechanical blockage. Esophageal manometry may also be useful in evaluating a motility disorder (e.g., achalasia) (Klinger and Strang 1987).

TABLE 6–1. Medical differential diagnosis of dysphagia

	Oropharyngeal	**Esophageal**
Neuromuscular	Multiple sclerosis	Achalasia
	Parkinson's disease	Diffuse esophageal spasm
	Postpolio syndrome (Sonies & Dalakasas, 1991)	Nutcracker esophagus
	Muscular dystrophy	
	Motor neuron disease (ALS)	
	Brain stem stroke	
Obstructive		Carcinoma
		Foreign body
		Esophageal webs
		Cervical osteoarthritis
Systemic	Thyrotoxicosis	Chagas' disease
	Sarcoidosis	
	Trichinosis	
Collagen	Polymyositis	Scleroderma
Vascular	Dermatomyositis	

Note. ALS = amyotrophic lateralizing sclerosis.
Source. Adapted from Epstein et al. 1993.

Epstein and colleagues (1993) outlined those esophageal disorders that are more pertinent to psychiatric medicine. These disorders generally involve abnormal esophageal motility. Chest discomfort when swallowing solids, difficulty ingesting liquids, heartburn, and regurgitation are typical in these cases (Reidel and Clouse 1985). "Nutcracker esophagus," a manometric pattern characterized by high-amplitude peristaltic contractions in the distal esophagus, has been described (Browning 1990). Experimental stressors have also been shown to increase esophageal activity resulting in these symptoms (Anderson et al. 1989). Anxiety that increases swallowing rates may also exacerbate existing esophageal disorders (Fonagu and Calloway 1986). Richter and colleagues (1986) identified personality profiles of patients with nutcracker esophagus that indicated susceptibility to gastrointestinal symptoms during emotional stress.

Individuals with esophagitis secondary to repeated contact with refluxed gastric and duodenal contents present clinically with heartburn, regurgitation, and retrosternal pain. Approximately 10% of the population will complain of heartburn at any one time (Wesdorp 1986). Psychiatric disorders are frequently observed with esophageal disorders (Bradley et al. 1990). Globus hystericus, or the sensation of a lump in the throat, has been associated with panic disorder and depression (Greenberg et al. 1988). Affective disorders and generalized anxiety commonly complicate disturbances of esophageal motility (Clouse and Lustman 1982). Individuals with a symptomatic hiatal hernia may also meet criteria for generalized anxiety or a depressive disorder (Nielzen et al. 1986). Interestingly, psychopharmacological and psychotherapeutic interventions for anxiety and depression can also ameliorate esophageal symptoms (Brown et al. 1986; Clouse et al. 1987).

Dyspepsia and Peptic Ulcer Disease

Dyspepsia, typically conceptualized as a stress response syndrome, is a generally accepted medical malady. Dyspepsia of unknown etiology accounts for some 30%–40% of cases of vague abdominal pain. Psychological factors that influence "gut" functioning, or dyspepsia, may be secondary to psychiatric illness (e.g., depression) (Drossman 1982). Others reported that dyspepsia results from excessive autonomic arousal, anxiety, or interpersonal problems in which anger is not expressed (Gomez and Dally 1977; Stockton et al. 1985; Talley et al. 1986). A report by E. A. Walker et al. (1992) alluded to the "high" prevalence rates of major depression, panic disorder, and agoraphobia among patients presenting to a tertiary care clinic with medically unexplained gastrointestinal symptoms. Interestingly, this report also analyzed structured psychiatric interviews of 18,571 subjects from the Epidemiologic Catchment Area study (Regier et al. 1984), noting that individuals with gastrointestinal symptoms when compared with those without symptoms experienced greater lifetime episodes of major depression (7.5% versus 2.9%), panic disorder (2.5% versus 0.7%), or agoraphobia (10% versus 3.6%).

Peptic ulcer disease (PUD), a general term applied to patients who have an ulcer (or have had one that has healed), has also been suspected of having a significant psychological origin. The corrosive action of gastric juice has been widely accepted as a contributing factor to the etiology of both dyspepsia and PUD since the mid-1800s (Gunzburg 1852). Thus, dyspepsia and PUD may both be associated with excessive vagal drive or excessive activity within gastrin-producing cells. These conditions may arise secondary to defective mucus protection of the lining of the gastrointestinal tract.

Our knowledge of the association between psychological factors and abdominal pain can be attributed to the observations of William Beaumont (1833), a Canadian surgeon who documented the correlation between anger and increased gastric fluid output by observing a gastric fistula in an injured Canadian lumberjack. General etiological factors in PUD include cigarette smoking, aspirin ingestion, and the use of corticosteroids. Alcohol has not been proven to cause ulcers; however, binge drinking causes gastritis, and individuals with alcoholic cirrhosis have an increased prevalence of ulcers. Both caffeinated and decaffeinated coffee stimulate acid secretion. Most research, however, has not indicated a relationship between coffee drinking and ulcers (Schubert 1984). Diet is no longer considered to be a factor in ulcer production.

The etiologies of gastric and duodenal ulcers differ. Duodenal ulcers may be associated with excessive secretion of hydrochloric acid by the stomach; delayed gastric emptying promotes gastric ulcers (Isenberg 1981). Duodenal ulcers occur more frequently in men, but there is no gender bias in gastric ulcers. Duodenal ulcers also occur more commonly in individuals with type O blood. Animal studies have provided a tentative link between brain chemistry and ulcer formation. For example, increased brain thyrotropin-releasing hormone synthesis may correlate with the presence of gastric ulcer.

PUD has been a primary focus of psychosomatic investigation. Early psychosomatic studies were hampered by imprecise definitions and lacked documentation of ulcer type and location. Alexander (1987) is best known for his psychosomatic hypothesis. He hypothesized that the patient with a duodenal ulcer has frustrated wishes to be loved and cared for that may result in persistent oral dependent needs. Weiner and colleagues (1957) investigated 2,073 army inductees by using psychological testing and serum pepsinogen levels, which correlated with basal rates of gastric acid secretion. In support of Alexander's theory, they found that the army inductees who later developed duodenal ulcers had high baseline pepsinogen levels and had intense dependency needs and conflicts with authority. These investigators thus integrated a somatic vulnerability with a vulnerable personality characteristic and a stressful life event (i.e., induction into the army). Similarly, emotional arousal, anxiety, and anger, in particular, are the psychophysiological causes of duodenal ulcer formation and are strongly associated with increased acid and pepsin secretion (Christensen 1988). The relationship between serum pepsinogen concentrations and other biobehavioral risk factors has been investigated. Personality features of hostility, irritability, hypersensitivity, and impaired coping ability (low ego strength) correlate significantly with serum pepsinogen concentration in ulcer patients $P \leq .005$) (P. Walker et al. 1988). Not unexpectedly, the incidence of cigarette smoking, alcohol intake, and aspirin ingestion is higher in ulcer patients *but* is not related to any coexistent psychopathology.

Alexander's (1987) inclusion of duodenal ulcer as a classic psychosomatic disorder does indeed appear reasonable when considering the above studies and noting that approximately 40% of duodenal ulcer patients relapse in the first year after medical treatment. Incidentally, psychological treatments continue to be recommended to these patients, especially in the management of stress, life-style factors, and anxiety. Chronic life stressors are known to predispose to the formation of duodenal ulcer and are correlated with symptomatic anxiety or depression. An analysis of 4,511 individuals 13 years after participating in the National Health and Nutrition Examination Survey revealed that peptic ulcers developed in 7.2% versus only 4.0% who perceived themselves as stressed—that is, 1.8 times more likely to develop ulcers when controlled for age, sex, education, smoking status, and aspirin use (Anda et al. 1992). Therefore, poor social support has been suggested as a possible risk factor for duodenal ulcer. However, evidence from the current literature does not definitively support the personality-related or psychosocial theories, nor does an association clearly exist between ulcer disease and Type A behavior or alexithymia. However, patients who relapse are often found to have coexisting anxiety or to have more frequent exposure to chronic stressors (Tennant 1988). PUD appears to be mediated potentially by a variety of psychological, behavioral, and physiological factors (Feldman et al. 1986; Walker et al. 1988). Data on the role of stress in the formation of PUD are far from uniform, and the results are often contradictory. The relationship between stress and psychosocial factors contributing to PUD is supported by discriminant analysis of patients with PUD versus control patients. The perception of negative impact of life events (although frequency of life events themselves did not differ), the number of relatives with PUD, and serum pepsinogen I concentration are also somewhat predictive.

Behavioral risk factors such as smoking, alcohol use, and aspirin ingestion are found, as previously mentioned, to be significantly higher in PUD patients. Systematic efforts to delineate a personality profile of these patients through the use of psychological testing procedures are lacking in the literature. Thus, regardless of personality type, the vulnerability and responsivity of an individual predisposed to developing PUD is presumably increased by situations that arouse anxiety, anger, or resentment and therefore elicit increased autonomic activity, which results in prolonged hypersecretion of the gastric mucosa (Williford et al. 1982).

Gilligan and colleagues (1987) reported that PUD was more common in divorced, separated, or widowed subjects. This case-controlled study implied that these subjects more frequently showed chronic personality difficulties that predisposed them to ulcer disease. Feldman and colleagues (1986) identified hypochondriasis, a negative perception of life events, dependency, and lowered ego strength as the four variables that might discriminate PUD patients from control subjects.

PUD either may be representative of a single disease entity or may be the result of a common pathogenic mechanism. There is an intriguing possibility that relevant psychological traits are genetically determined (Magni et al. 1986). Perhaps specific personality profiles are associated with a predisposition to ulcer disease, but an etiological relationship has yet to be confirmed. Evidence indicates genetic and familial factors that influence development of a duodenal ulcer and increased acid-pepsin secretion in individuals exposed to a variety of stressful stimuli (Williford et al. 1982). Interestingly, decreasing prevalence of both gastric and duodenal ulcers is currently well established, and a clear familial incidence has been documented in the literature (Wolf 1985). The literature frequently describes patients with dyspepsia and ulcers who have characteristic personality traits (i.e., dependent, compulsive, or avoidant). A consensus on the personality and psychological aspects related to chronic dyspepsia or PUD is reflected in the literature (i.e., patients who more typically present with psychological problems of dependence or independence also possess high levels of anxiety) (Epstein et al. 1993). Langeluddecke and colleagues (1990) carefully examined the association of psychological factors in a group of patients with duodenal ulcers and a matched dyspepsia group. The dyspepsia patients had significantly more symptoms of anxiety and tension and higher scores for trait tension and hostility than the peptic ulcer group. Magni and colleagues (1987) demonstrated that both dyspepsia and PUD were associated with a higher prevalence of psychiatric diagnoses than that observed in control subjects (86.7% versus 25.0%, respectively); anxiety disorders occurred with the highest incidence (66.7%). Their study of psychiatric disturbances revealed that Type A behavior associated with hostility, a chronic sense of time urgency, and competitiveness were much more likely to be associated with PUD. Tennant and colleagues (1986) studied psychological correlates of gastric and duodenal ulcer disease and noted that the two diagnostic groups did not differ significantly on measures of trait anxiety, tension, introversion, or Type A behavior.

Whether psychological factors or psychiatric disorders per se contribute to the onset or chronicity of nonulcer dyspepsia, as well as duodenal ulcer, remains controversial. Although psychological testing has not established a clearly defined personality type in the etiology of these disorders, the inability to express emotion (alexithymia), which may result in excessive autonomic arousal, may have etiological significance (Stoudemire 1991). However, individuals with dyspepsia who present for investigation or participate in studies are unlikely to repress emotional reactions consciously (Talley et al. 1988). By contrast, an animal study of emotionality and stress-induced ulcers in rats investigated electrophysiological activity in the central amygdaloid nucleus in these animals (Henke 1988). The investigators concluded that activity in the central nucleus of the amygdala reflects certain emotional characteristics of rats and is associated with the susceptibility to stress-induced ulcers.

The majority of duodenal and gastric ulcers will likely heal without intervention, but clinical intervention may enhance the therapeutic process. Clinical experience also suggests that stress is frequently the more relevant contributory factor in the exacerbation of PUD. Psychological and behavioral factors are generally believed to be important in some forms of PUD but perhaps not in others. Consideration of psychiatric treatment should therefore be based on the individual's psychological characteristics and not solely on the presence of PUD (Feldman 1980). Chapell and colleagues (1936) used dietary management and group therapy with an educational component similar to Buchanan's (1978) two-step methodology for the group treatment of patients with organic illnesses. This favorable method allowed group members to learn about the physiological aspects of their gastrointestinal disease in a formal didactic fashion. The treated group had greater improvement than did untreated control subjects. This outcome is consistent with prior reports involving the application of stress management training, relaxation therapy, and assertiveness training, which are all purported to be effective in diminishing ulcerative pain and in reducing antacid ingestion (Brooks and Richardson 1980).

Inflammatory Bowel Disease

Inflammatory bowel disease refers to two processes: ulcerative colitis and regional enteritis (Crohn's disease) (Farmer 1981). Ulcerative colitis is generally limited to the mucosal lining of the large intestine. Its dominant symptoms are diarrhea and hematochezia. In severe disease states, the individual will develop multiple watery stools that can lead to dehydration and anemia. Crohn's disease is a transmural process that may affect any part of the alimentary canal but most often involves the distal ileum and proximal colon. Intestinal obstruction, fistulas, and abscesses may occur, resulting in symptoms such as abdominal pain, fever, and severe weight loss. Ulcerative colitis increases the risk of colonic cancer to a greater extent than does Crohn's disease. Crohn's disease may recur relentlessly despite long periods of apparent remission, whereas ulcerative colitis can actually be cured by colectomy.

Ulcerative colitis predominantly affects a younger population, the greatest incidence occurring between ages 15 and 20 years. The diagnosis is associated with significant chronic disability and predisposes the individual to an unusually high incidence of carcinoma of the colon. Psychological impact is significant for both patients and their families; surgery is often necessary when severe or prolonged symptoms of rectal bleeding, diarrhea, weight loss, extracolonic manifestations, and abdominal pain occur. When the illness is chronic and unremitting, it is characterized by exacerbations and remissions, often without regard or response to the medical treatment.

Inflammatory bowel diseases remain a mystery with respect to their etiology and the role of psychological factors. A variety of psychological factors may indeed affect the course of ulcerative colitis. Clinical research has considered both autoimmune and infectious factors as contributing to the etiology and pathogenesis of ulcerative colitis. Mucosal lesions found in ulcerative colitis patients have been documented to persist for years after the onset of the disease regardless of whether symptoms are present. This latter observation may explain the concomitant nature of psychological and emotional reactions. Incidentally, patients with ulcerative colitis are no more likely to have current or lifetime psychiatric diagnoses than are medically ill control patients (Helzer et al. 1982).

Despite the early literature identifying ulcerative colitis as a psychosomatic disease, this etiological concept must be strongly questioned. Ulcerative colitis has been the subject of many psychosocial studies of personality, intrapsychic conflicts, and categories of life events presumably associated with the onset, exacerbation, and remission of the disease. However, many of the methodological problems in the literature leave doubt as to the significance of personality or psychological and behavioral patterns associated with ulcerative colitis (North et al. 1990). Studies have consistently alluded to the presence of compulsive personalities in a parental figure, especially the mother. Traits of perfectionism, neatness, orderliness, obstinacy, conformism, and punctuality are often mentioned. Many of these patients are stereotyped as being dependent and immature and may be described as infantile and regressed (Rosenbaum 1985). Similarly, numerous anecdotal clinical reports of ulcerative colitis patients have examined patterns of infantile, dependent behavior and eroded self-esteem and confidence. North and colleagues reviewed the English language literature for associations between psychiatric factors and the development of ulcerative colitis. Virtually all studies cited had methodological flaws. This review concurred with other reports (Andrews et al. 1987; Tarter et al. 1987) in which it was evident that the well-controlled studies did not establish an association between ulcerative colitis and psychopathology.

Specific therapeutic strategies for the management of psychological influences that potentially affect the course of ulcerative colitis are also not well established or substantiated. Unfortunately, approximately one-third of ulcerative colitis patients require surgical treatment. Many of these individuals do not seek or receive further general medical or psychiatric care and are then followed by their surgeon. Thus, the surgeon may assume the role of primary care physician, a role for which he or she may not be well prepared. Perhaps clinical management and future studies might best include a consulting psychiatrist or psychologist who could continue to assess the patient and maintain a liaison with the surgeon.

Ulcerative colitis must be differentiated on psychological grounds from Crohn's disease. E. A. Walker and colleagues (1990b) noted that multiple surgical procedures are more likely with Crohn's disease than with ulcerative colitis. Consequently, patients with Crohn's disease may have a higher prevalence of secondary illness. Essential differences between Crohn's disease and ulcerative colitis must be understood in providing psychological support for these patients. Specifically, the individual with Crohn's disease will have to cope with an uncertain and relentless disease that has exacerbations and remissions. The relatively favorable prognosis of the ulcerative colitis patient after colectomy stands in great contrast to that of the Crohn's disease patient, whose illness may persist. In one study, the three more prominent concerns of inflammatory bowel disease patients were 1) having an ostomy bag, 2) their energy level, and 3) the possibility of having surgery. Patients with Crohn's disease were significantly more concerned with pain, whereas the typical ulcerative colitis patient was significantly more concerned with loss of bowel control and development of cancer (Drossman et al. 1989). Therefore, psychological treatment must be directed toward coping with specific life stressors, with problems including the actual treatment itself, and with the existential nature of the chronic disease (Zisook and DeVaul 1977).

Contemporary investigators have continued the attempt to distinguish psychological factors in Crohn's disease from those found in ulcerative colitis. Whybrow and colleagues (1968) noted a variety of noxious life changes that could potentially exacerbate active episodes of Crohn's disease. Of these, depressive symptoms were often described with a more lengthy illness. Two controlled studies (Helzer et al. 1982, 1984) that utilized structured interviews and operational diagnostic criteria suggest that ulcerative colitis patients are no more likely than medically ill control patients to have psychiatric diagnoses. Crohn's disease patients, however, show significantly higher prevalence of depression than do control subjects. Interestingly, the severity of gastrointestinal symptoms and psychiatric symptoms are independent; there is no consistent temporal sequence of involvement.

McKegney and colleagues (1970) also compared ulcerative colitis with Crohn's disease but reported no significant differences between groups from psychosocial, psychiatric, or behavioral perspectives. However, patients with more severe physical disabilities displayed more depressive symptoms. Similarly, Andrews and colleagues (1987), using a self-report measure and the Structured Clinical Interview for DSM-III-R, found that physical illness in Crohn's disease was indeed associated with psychiatric morbidity; the same association was not significant for ulcerative colitis patients. Tarter and colleagues (1987) reported that patients with Crohn's disease, compared with control subjects, demonstrated a significantly greater prevalence of anxiety and depression as measured by the Diagnostic Interview Schedule. Again, ulcerative colitis patients did not have an excessive prevalence of any psychiatric disorder.

Irritable Bowel Syndrome

The more frequently documented gastroenterological syndrome related to psychiatric influences is irritable bowel syndrome (IBS). IBS is a heterogeneous condition of uncertain etiology that accounts for 50% of ambulatory cases seen by gastroenterologists (Thompson 1979). The syndrome is comprised of a cluster of bowel symptoms, including alternating diarrhea, constipation, and abdominal pain. IBS may be partitioned into diarrhea-predominant, constipation-predominant, and mixed varieties. Classification of this disorder is difficult. A variety of investigations have shown that "normal" patient populations frequently report bowel habits similar to those of patients with operationally defined IBS (Thompson and Heaton 1980). Prevalence figures range from 13% to 20% (E. A. Walker et al. 1990a). Psychological criteria are not well defined, but psychiatric disturbances are widely reported (North et al.

1990). IBS is usually defined by abdominal pain and change in bowel habit, either diarrhea or constipation, that occur in the absence of abnormalities on physical examination and laboratory diagnostic tests.

The etiology and physiology of IBS are not fully understood. IBS is presumably associated with disturbances in motility that are influenced by psychological factors found in symptomatic patients whose symptoms tend to recur in a chronic, relapsing, and remitting course. Noncolonic gastrointestinal symptoms are often present in IBS, probably because motility disturbances may be seen throughout the gastrointestinal tract. Extragastrointestinal symptoms are common as well (Whorwell 1989). One study (Young et al. 1976) found that 28% of patients met criteria for somatization disorder. Most investigators would agree that IBS involves a combination of psychological and physiological factors.

Several terms have been used interchangeably with IBS, and a more distinct diagnostic nosology has been evolving. Several systematic studies (Latimer 1979; Latimer et al. 1981; Whitehead et al. 1980) identified possible psychological characteristics of such patients. The evidence suggests that patients with IBS are more often psychologically disturbed compared, in a controlled fashion, with the general population, and compared with individuals suffering from other medical conditions. Psychological stress as a consequence of stressful life events was significantly correlated to disability days and number of medical clinic visits in a group of 383 women with IBS (Whitehead et al. 1992). Those subjects who satisfied restrictive diagnostic criteria for IBS were compared with a group with abdominal pain without IBS and control subjects without bowel dysfunction. This irritable bowel group showed significantly greater reactivity to stress using regression analysis. No distinctive personality profile exists for IBS patients; however, anxiety is believed to play an important role. Also, it is well established that IBS individuals have a greater than 70% incidence of psychological, behavioral, or psychiatric disorders; have a large proportion of unrecognized psychiatric disturbances; represent a heterogeneous group in terms of psychiatric disorders; and are more commonly diagnosed in teaching hospitals (Latimer 1985). A comprehensive review by E. A. Walker and colleagues (1990b) outlined many other clinical features of IBS that are beyond the scope of this chapter.

If IBS is a condition in which the gut is hypersensitive and hyperactive to mechanical and chemical stimuli, it may be comparable with asthma in the respiratory system (Read 1987). The psychophysiological disturbances found with IBS suggest that an underlying biological predisposition toward the abnormality exists. Studies report abnormal electrical rhythms in the smooth muscle of the rectum and rectosigmoid colon as well as rectal and colonic motor hyperactivity during baseline recordings and during rectal distension following food intake or the injection of neostigmine. These laboratory findings have frequently been replicated. In one study of IBS (Whitehead et al. 1980), physiological and psychological differences were examined by comparing diarrhea-predominant and constipation-predominant patients. Patients with these differing profiles of IBS were compared with control subjects to determine whether subtypes of IBS could be distinguished based on colonic motility or psychological test scores. A provocative test involving stepwise distension of the rectosigmoidal area revealed two types of colonic motility: slow and fast. Slow contractions having durations of at least 15 seconds and occurring at irregular intervals were more frequent in IBS patients than in control subjects patients but did not differentiate constipation from diarrhea. Fast contractions having durations of less than 15 seconds and occurring in runs at frequencies of 6–9 cpm were more frequent in patients with diarrhea than in control subjects or constipated IBS patients. Constipated patients showed no more fast contractions than control subjects.

Other studies (Wise 1986) have also suggested that individuals with IBS may have abnormal myoelectric activity of the colon, abnormalities of gastric hormones, and food allergies. Environmental stress, life events, and psychological factors are now known to be associated with changes in colonic physiology (E. A. Walker et al. 1990b). Based on data from studies already mentioned, there is a consensus among investigators that there is a colonic abnormality that is indeed peculiar to IBS patients. Therefore, any study of IBS must include a control group consisting of subjects who are equally disturbed psychologically but who do not have the prototypical abnormal bowel symptoms. For example, elevated levels of anxiety, interpersonal sensitivity, depression, hostility, and somatization of affect have been noted among both groups. No significant trait differences have been demonstrated between patients with diarrhea and those with constipation. However, a report has suggested the clinical utility and greater psychometric sensitivity of the Hopkins Symptom Checklist in comparison with the Minnesota Multiphasic Personality Inventory to measure the behavioral profiles of patients with constipation (Wald et al. 1992). Two studies (Drossman et al. 1988; Whitehead et al. 1988) indicated that whereas "patients" with IBS have psychological problems, "nonpatients" who meet IBS criteria do not. Barsky (1987) opined that IBS is best described as a dimensional rather than a categorical illness. A comprehensive review by Epstein and colleagues (1993) further noted that perhaps patients with IBS simply overestimate their excretory problems and seek medical care because of abnormal illness behavior.

Psychological factors may indeed be more relevant in IBS patients who develop abdominal and psychiatric symptoms simultaneously, in which case treatment of the latter may relieve the bowel symptoms. Also, psychiatric disorders may precipitate increased concern about bowel symptoms resulting in patient presentation to the gastroenterology clinic for evaluation of chronic mild symptoms. Higher prevalence of psychopathology is observed among patient populations with IBS (Sandler et al. 1984). Johnsen and colleagues (1986) reported a strong association between IBS and psychiatric disturbance (i.e., depression, insomnia, problems of coping, or the use and abuse of analgesics). However, life-style, dietary habits, and social variables did not reveal an association with IBS. A weak negative association was shown between age and the prevalence of reported pain in IBS. Women reported abdominal symptoms, especially cramping abdominal pain, significantly more often than did men. Illness behavior was believed to be particularly pertinent in these cases and was more significant than a simple response to the abdominal symptoms. Patients possessing chronic, neurotic symptoms as part of their illness behavior were likely to present with coexistent organic disease, especially if new-onset bowel symptoms were present. Not unexpectedly, these patients were found to be at high risk for becoming persistent clinic attenders.

Social learning may also contribute to the etiology of IBS when contrasted to PUD (Whitehead et al. 1982). Assessment of IBS patients has consistently revealed a high prevalence of psychological symptoms compared with nonpsychiatric patients and healthy control groups. Lowman and colleagues (1987) analyzed childhood events of adult patients who suffered from IBS. IBS patients differed from control patients by reporting more severe bowel problems, more frequent doctor visits in childhood, and more pain associated with current bowel symptoms. The study also showed that IBS patients had greater parental attention to illness with more frequent school absences and doctor visits than control patients. Loss and separation were the key psychodynamic issues among IBS patients during childhood. Conflicted or dependent maternal relationships with the children were also more frequently reported among married IBS patients than control patients (Lowman et al. 1987). These family constellation factors may therefore contribute significantly to the development of IBS.

IBS patients have an increased incidence of psychological disturbances compared with patients who suffer from inflammatory bowel disease (E. A. Walker et al. 1990a; Young et al. 1976). Psychiatric illness may precede the onset of gastrointestinal symptoms (E. A. Walker et al. 1990a). Such studies suggest that psychological illness is associated with the IBS and is not merely a reaction to the discomfort of symptoms (for an excellent review, see E. A. Walker and colleagues 1990a). IBS patients are more anxious and depressed than control patients and tend to overuse medical services (Camilleri and Neri 1989).

A strong and consistent association between functional abdominal disorders and psychological factors suggests the need for psychological interventions other than just prescribing drugs or diets. Stress alone does not appear to be associated with symptomatic IBS unless provoked by an anxiety state (Ford et al. 1987). Arapakis and colleagues (1986) compared IBS and ulcerative colitis patients; both experimental groups were found to be less assertive, more intropunitive, more anxious, and more depressed than control patients. IBS patients, however, were more assertive and less intropunitive than ulcerative colitis patients. Both ulcerative colitis and IBS patients were found to be psychologically distressed and used neurotic defense mechanisms. Also, more IBS patients had premorbid psychiatric symptoms than control patients and ulcerative colitis comparison patients.

IBS patients (compared with PUD or dyspepsia patients) have always shown the personality features, or the same consistency, as was noted with PUD. However, IBS patients have generally been regarded as more neurotic and depressed. Sjödin and Svedlund (1985) studied 101 IBS and 103 PUD patients; their overall results revealed that mental symptoms and personality profiles were essentially the same in IBS and PUD, and both groups differed from a control population. The combination of medical treatment with psychotherapy improved the outcome for both IBS and PUD subgroups.

Because the role of stress and personality factors in IBS remains unclear (Camilleri and Neri 1989), the symptoms of IBS are perhaps better conceptualized as a subset of a broader problem that may meet DSM-III-R (American Psychiatric Association 1987) criteria for a particular mood, anxiety, somatoform, or adjustment disorder. Clearly, more research using systematic diagnostic criteria is needed to clarify which psychological abnormalities might play a role in the etiology of IBS, when they are merely coincidental, and when the psychiatric disorder (personality disorder) leads to illness behavior (Clouse 1988). A number of considerations have been found in this regard. First, the measurement of psychological factors has generally been imprecise. Second, most studies consider IBS patients as a single group without making allowances for differing symptom patterns. Third, conclusions have been drawn about hospital samples and extrapolated to all IBS subjects without taking into account factors that affect consulting behavior (Creed and Guthrie 1987). Recent experiments that examine the gastrointestinal response to acute stress and amplify prior investigations confirm that central stimuli, via emotional stress, can indeed produce measurable gastrointestinal changes. These changes are not uniformly predictable based on knowledge of the control mechanisms alone. Thus, laboratory experiments cannot be directly extrapolated to psychological and behavioral factors and their relationship to IBS and other gastrointestinal conditions. Moreover, there are few physiological studies of the more chronic disorders.

Although they are scarce, reports of psychiatric interventions for IBS patients suggest that a treatment plan that includes supportive psychotherapy or hypnotherapy may be beneficial. However, the long-term efficacy of such treatments remains questionable (Langeluddecke 1985). Various treatments have been used for IBS (Wise 1986). These include dietary management, anticholinergic medications, and use of anxiolytics or tricyclic antidepressants (Lydiard et al. 1986; Noyes et al. 1990). The usual therapeutic strategy for treatment of IBS patients employs a variety of combined psychiatric-nonpsychiatric medical therapies, including education, symptom management, stress management, and contingency management and pharmacotherapy for anxiety, depression, and other relevant psychiatric symptoms.

Irritable bowel complaints may respond to antidepressants or anxiolytics whether or not the patient is clinically depressed. Buspirone, which has been shown to have both antidepressant and anxiolytic effects with minimal side effects, may prove to be extremely helpful in this population (Richter et al. 1986). Brief psychotherapy or combined cognitive-behavioral therapy and/or behavioral techniques may also benefit the patient (Wise et al. 1982). A biopsychosocial perspective that addresses multigenerational family patterns of anxiety, depression, and somatization in the context of stress may also provide some basis for understanding and treating symptomatic IBS patients (Crouch 1988). A thorough review of this approach may be found elsewhere (Epstein et al. 1993).

Discussion

Knowledge of the psychological and behavioral factors that may influence gastrointestinal disease is far from conclusive. However, factors identified by the more recent reports cited in this chapter and the implications for a psychiatric approach to gastrointestinal patients are quite relevant. The role of psychological factors influencing gastrointestinal conditions are noteworthy for the following: 1) psychiatric disturbances (i.e., anxiety, depression, or somatization); 2) behavioral reactions, including the abuse of alcohol, drugs, and tobacco; 3) noncompliance or resistance to prevention therapy; and 4) various responses to intervention. Relevant, specific physiological or psychophysiological reactions may also be mediated through neuroendocrine, immunological, or other psychobiological systems. Obviously, these systems and their relevance in gastroenterological dysfunction are worthy of further research.

Gastrointestinal conditions must therefore continue to be considered in the context of psychological or behavioral factors simultaneously. Of particular importance are psychosocial stressors (precipitants), psychological influences on well-being, and modifiers of outcome from therapeutic interventions. Other important variables, the subject of current studies, include the relative influence of coping abilities and the significance of social support. Research has begun to examine the following:

1) personality factors; 2) psychological factors; 3) stressful life events and their relationship to the physical condition together with possible interactions among biological parameters, the central nervous system, and psychosocial parameters; and 4) psychiatric disorders. Personality factors, especially those involving dependence-independence problems, high levels of anxiety, or depression, are frequently observed in gastroenterology patient populations. However, a number of studies suggesting a role for psychological factors need to be replicated or carried out with larger numbers of patients and improved methodology. Thus, the relationship, association, and interaction among psychological factors and gastrointestinal maladies remain areas in need of future research.

Any new investigation of the psychological and behavioral aspects of gastrointestinal disorders (particularly those focusing on etiology and pathophysiology) will undoubtedly benefit from diagnostic rigor. Improved sampling, methodology, and selection of patients and better use of controls may also clarify the heterogeneity of these gastroenterological disorders. Common denominators in the etiology of psychosocially or behaviorally induced gastrointestinal disorders may also enable some generalization and application to other medical conditions. Finally, factors that are more likely to exacerbate, perpetuate, or significantly affect the course of an illness may then be clarified further (or better delineated), particularly as the nosological approach evolves.

References

Alexander F: Psychosomatic Medicine: Its Principles and Applications. New York, WW Norton, 1987

American Psychiatric Association: Diagnostic and Statistical Manual of Mental Disorders, 3rd Edition, Revised. Washington, DC, American Psychiatric Association, 1987

American Psychiatric Association: Diagnostic and Statistical Manual of Mental Disorders, 4th Edition. Washington, DC, American Psychiatric Association, 1994

Anda RF, Williamson DF, Escobedo LG, et al: Self perceived stress and the risk of peptic ulcer disease: a longitudinal study of US adults. Arch Intern Med 152:829–833, 1992

Anderson KO, Dalton CB, Bradley LA, et al: Stress induces alteration of esophageal pressures in healthy volunteers and non-cardiac chest pain patients. Dig Dis Sci 34:83–91, 1989

Andrews H, Barczak P, Allan RN: Psychiatric illness in patients with inflammatory bowel disease. Gut 28:1600–1604, 1987

Arapakis G, Lyketsos CG, Gerolymatos K, et al: Low dominance and high intropunitiveness in ulcerative colitis and irritable bowel syndrome. Psychother Psychosom 46:171–176, 1986

Barsky AJ: Investigating the psychological aspects of the irritable bowel syndrome (editorial). Gastroenterology 93:902–904, 1987

Beaumont W: Experiments and Observations on the Gastric Juice and Physiology of Digestion. Plattsburg, NY, FP Allen, 1833

Bradley LA, McDonald JE, Richter JE: Psychophysiological interactions in the esophageal diseases: implications for assessment and treatment. Seminars in Gastrointestinal Disease 1:5–22, 1990

Brooks GR, Richardson FC: Emotional skills training: a treatment program for duodenal ulcer. Behav Res Ther 11:198–207, 1980

Brown SR, Schwartz JM, Sumergrad P, et al: Globus hystericus syndrome responsive to antidepressants. Am J Psychiatry 143:917–918, 1986

Browning TH, Members of the Patient Care Committee of the American Gastroenterological Association: Diagnosis of chest pain of esophageal origin. Dig Dis Sci 35:289–293, 1990

Buchanan DC: Group therapy for chronically physically ill patients. Psychosomatics 19:425–431, 1978

Camilleri M, Neri M: Motility disorders and stress. Dig Dis Sci 34:1777–1786, 1989

Chapell MN, Stefano JJ, Rogerson JS, et al: The value of group psychological procedures in the treatment of peptic ulcer. American Journal of Digestive Diseases 3:813–817, 1936

Christensen NJ: Psychosocial stress and catecholamines: their relationship to aging, duodenal ulcer, hypochondriasis and hypertension. Pharmacol Toxicol 63 (suppl 1):24–26, 1988

Clouse RE: Anxiety and gastrointestinal illness. Psychiatr Clin North Am 11:399–517, 1988

Clouse RE, Lustman PJ: Psychiatric illnesses and contraction abnormalities of the esophagus. N Engl J Med 309:1337–1342, 1982

Clouse RE, Lustman PJ, Eckert TC, et al: Low-dose trazodone for symptomatic patients with esophageal contraction abnormalities. Gastroenterology 92:1027–1036, 1987

Creed F, Guthrie E: Psychological factors in the irritable bowel syndrome. Gut 28:1307–1318, 1987

Crouch MA: Irritable bowel syndrome: toward a biopsychosocial systems understanding. Prim Care 15:99–110, 1988

Drossman DA: Patients with psychogenic abdominal pain: six years observation in the medical setting. Am J Psychiatry 139:1549–1557, 1982

Drossman DA, McKee DC, Sandler RS, et al: Psychosocial factors in the irritable bowel syndrome. Gastroenterology 95:701–708, 1988

Drossman DA, Patrick DL, Mitchell CM, et al: Health-related quality of life in inflammatory bowel disease. Dig Dis Sci 34:1379–1386, 1989

Drossman DA, Leserman J, Nachman G, et al: Sexual and physical abuse in women with functional or organic gastrointestinal disorders. Ann Intern Med 113:828–833, 1990

Epstein SA, Wise TN, Goldberg RL: Gastroenterology, in Psychiatric Care of the Medical Patient. Edited by Stoudemire A, Fogel BS. New York, Oxford University Press, 1993, pp 611–625

Farmer RG: Factors in long term prognosis of patients with inflammatory bowel disease. Am J Gastroenterol 75:97–109, 1981

Feldman EJ: Psychosomatic factors in duodenal ulcer disease. Brain Res Bull 1:39–42, 1980

Feldman M, Walker P, Green JL, et al: Life events stress and psychosocial factors in men with peptic ulcer disease. Gastroenterology 91:1370–1379, 1986

Fonagu P, Calloway SP: The effect of emotional arousal on spontaneous swallowing rates. J Psychosom Res 30:183–188, 1986

Ford MJ, Miller PM, Eastwood J, et al: Life events, psychiatric illness and the irritable bowel syndrome. Gut 28:160–165, 1987

Gilligan I, Fung L, Piper DW, et al: Life event stress and chronic difficulties in duodenal ulcer: a case control study. J Psychosom Res 31:117–123, 1987

Gomez J, Dally P: Psychologically medicated abdominal pain in surgical and medical outpatient clinics. BMJ 1:1451–1453, 1977

Greenberg DB, Stern TA, Weilburg JB: The fear of choking: three successfully treated cases. Psychosomatics 29:126–129, 1988

Gunzburg F: Zur Kritik des Magenschweres, insbesondere des Perforirenden. Archiv fur physiologiche Heilkunde 11:516–527, 1852

Helzer JE, Stillings WA, Channas S, et al: A controlled study of the association between ulcerative colitis and psychiatric diagnosis. Dig Dis Sci 27:513–518, 1982

Helzer JE, Channas S, Norland CC, et al: A study of the association between Crohn's disease and psychiatric illness. Gastroenterology 86:324–330, 1984

Henke PG: Electrophysiological activity in the central nucleus of the amygdala: emotionality and stress ulcers in rats. Behav Neurosci 102:77–83, 1988

Isenberg JI: Peptic ulcer. Disease-A-Month 28:1–58, 1981

Johnsen R, Jacobsen BK, Forde OH: Associations between symptoms of irritable colon and psychological and social conditions and lifestyle. BMJ 292:1633–1635, 1986

Katon W: Panic disorder and somatization. Am J Med 77:101–106, 1984

Klinger RL, Strang JP: Psychiatric aspects of swallowing disorders. Psychosomatics 28:572–576, 1987

Langeluddecke PM: Psychological aspects of irritable bowel syndrome. Aust N Z J Psychiatry 19:218–226, 1985

Langeluddecke P, Goulston K, Tennant C: Psychological factors in dyspepsia of unknown cause: a comparison with peptic ulcer disease. J Psychosom Res 34:215–222, 1990

Latimer P: Psychophysiologic disorders: a critical appraisal of concept and theory illustrated with reference to the irritable bowel syndrome (IBS). Psychol Med 9:71–80, 1979

Latimer PR: Irritable bowel syndrome, in Psychosomatic Illness Review. Edited by Dorfman W, Cristofar L. New York, Macmillan, 1985, pp 61–75

Latimer P, Sarna S, Campbell D, et al: Colonic motor and myoelectrical activity: a comparative study of normal subjects, psychoneurotic patients, and patients with irritable bowel syndrome. Gastroenterology 80:893–901, 1981

Lowman BC, Drossman DA, Cramer RE, et al: Recollection of childhood events in adults with irritable bowel syndrome. J Clin Gastroenterol 9:324–330, 1987

Lydiard RB, Laraia MT, Howell EF, et al: Can panic disorder present as irritable bowel syndrome? J Clin Psychiatry 47:470–473, 1986

Magni G, DiMario F, Aggio L, et al: Psychosomatic factors and peptic ulcer disease. Hepatogastroenterology 33:131–137, 1986

Magni G, DiMario F, Borgherini G, et al: Personality and duodenal ulcer response to antisecretory treatment. Digestion 38:152–155, 1987

McKegney FP, Gordon RO, Levine SM: A psychosomatic comparison of patients with ulcerative colitis and Crohn's disease. Psychosom Med 32:153–166, 1970

Nielzen S, Pettersson KI, Regnel G, et al: The role of psychiatric factors in symptoms of hiatus hernia or gastric reflux. Acta Psychiatr Scand 73:214–220, 1986

North CS, Clouse RE, Spitznagel EL, et al: The relation of ulcerative colitis to psychiatric factors: a review of findings and methods. Am J Psychiatry 147:974–981, 1990

Noyes R, Cook B, Garvey M, et al: Reduction of gastrointestinal symptoms following treatment for panic disorder. Psychosomatics 31:75–79, 1990

Read NW: Irritable bowel syndrome (IBS)—definition and pathophysiology. Scand J Gastroenterol Suppl 130:7–13, 1987

Regier DA, Myers JK, Kramer M, et al: The NIMH Epidemiologic Catchment Area program: historical context, major objectives, and study populations characteristics. Arch Gen Psychiatry 41:934–941, 1984

Reidel WL, Clouse RE: Variations in clinical presentation of patients with esophageal contraction abnormalities. Dig Dis Sci 30:1065–1071, 1985

Richter JE, Obrecht WF, Bradley LA, et al: Psychological similarities between patients with the nutcracker esophagus and irritable bowel syndrome. Dig Dis Sci 31:131–138, 1986

Rosenbaum M: Ulcerative colitis, in Psychosomatic Illness Review. Edited by Dorfman W, Cristofar L. New York, Macmillan, 1985, pp 76–89

Sandler RS, Drossman DA, Nathan HP, et al: Symptom complaints and health care seeking behavior in subjects with bowel dysfunction. Gastroenterology 87:314–318, 1984

Schubert TT: Update in treatment of peptic ulcer disease. Mo Med 11:723–727, 1984

Sjödin I, Svedlund J: Psychological aspects of non-ulcer dyspepsia: a psychosomatic view focusing on a comparison between the irritable bowel syndrome and peptic ulcer disease. Scand J Gastroenterol Suppl 109:51–58, 1985

Stockton M, Weinman J, McColl I: An investigation of psychosocial factors in patients with upper abdominal pain: a comparison with other groups of surgical outpatients. J Psychosom Res 29:191–198, 1985

Stoudemire A: Somatothymia, parts I and II. Psychosomatics 32:365–381, 1991

Switz DM: What the gastroenterologist does all day: a survey of a state societies practice. Gastroenterology 70:1048–1050, 1976

Talley NJ, Fung LH, Gilligan IJ, et al: Association of anxiety, neuroticism, and depression with dyspepsia of unknown cause. Gastroenterology 90:886–892, 1986

Talley NJ, Ellard K, Jones M, et al: Suppression of emotions in essential dyspepsia and chronic duodenal ulcer: a case-control study. Scan J Gastroenterol 23:337–340, 1988

Tarter RE, Switala J, Carra J, et al: Inflammatory bowel disease: psychiatric status of patients before and after disease onset. Int J Psychiatry Med 17:173–181, 1987

Tennant C: Psychosocial causes of duodenal ulcer. Aust N Z J Psychiatry 22:195–201, 1988

Tennant C, Goulston K, Langeluddecke P: Psychological correlates of gastric and duodenal ulcer disease. Psychol Med 16:365–371, 1986

Thompson WG: The Irritable Gut. Baltimore, MD, University Park, 1979

Thompson WG, Heaton KW: Functional bowel disorders in apparently healthy people. Gastroenterology 79:283–288, 1980

Van Valkenburg C, Winokur G, Behar D, et al: Depressed women with panic attacks. J Clin Psychiatry 45:367–369, 1984

Wald A, Burgio K, Holeva K, et al: Psychological evaluation of patients with severe idiopathic constipation: which instrument to use. Am J Gastroenterology 87:977–980, 1992

Walker EA, Roy-Byrne PP, Katon WJ: Irritable bowel syndrome and psychiatric illness. Am J Psychiatry 147:565–572, 1990a

Walker EA, Roy-Byrne PP, Katon WJ, et al: Psychiatric illness and irritable bowel syndrome: a comparison with inflammatory bowel disease. Am J Psychiatry 147:1656–1661, 1990b

Walker EA, Katon WJ, Jemelka RP, et al: Comorbidity of gastrointestinal complaints, depression and anxiety in the Epidemiologic Catchment Area Study. Am J Med 92 (suppl 1A):26S–30S, 1992

Walker P, Luther J, Samloff IM, et al: Life events stress and psychosocial factors in men with peptic ulcer disease, II: relationships with serum pepsinogen concentrations and behavioral risk factors. Gastroenterology 94:323–330, 1988

Weiner H, Thaler M, Reiser MF, et al: Etiology of duodenal ulcer, I: relation of specific psychological characteristics to rate of gastric secretion (serum pepsinogen) (abstract). Psychosom Med 19:1, 1957

Wesdorp ICE: Reflux esophagitis: a review. Postgrad Med J 62 (suppl 2):43–55, 1986

Whitehead WE, Bosmajian L, Zonderman AB, et al: Symptoms of psychologic distress associated with irritable bowel syndrome. Gastroenterology 95:709–714, 1988

Whitehead WE, Engel BT, Schuster MM: Irritable bowel syndrome: physiological and psychological differences between diarrhea-predominant and constipation-predominant patients. Dig Dis Sci 25:404–413, 1980

Whitehead WE, Winget C, Fedoravicius AS, et al: Learned illness behavior in patients with irritable bowel syndrome and peptic ulcer. Dig Dis Sci 27:202–208, 1982

Whitehead WE, Crowell MD, Robinson JC, et al: Effects of stressful life events on bowel symptoms: subjects with irritable bowel syndrome compared with subjects without bowel dysfunction. Gut 33:825–830, 1992

Whorwell PJ: Diagnosis and management of irritable bowel syndrome: discussion paper. J R Soc Med 82:613–614, 1989

Whybrow PC, Kane TJ, Lipton MA: Regional ileitis and psychiatric disorders (letter). Psychosom Med 30:209, 1968

Williford DJ, Ormsbee HS, Norman W: Hind-brain GABA receptors influence parasympathetic outflow to the stomach. Science 214:193–194, 1982

Wise TN: Psychological management of IBS. Practical Gastroenterology 10:40–50, 1986

Wise TN, Cooper JN, Ahmed S: The efficacy of group therapy for patients with irritable bowel syndrome. Psychosomatics 23:465–469, 1982

Wolf S: Peptic ulcer, in Psychosomatic Illness Review. Edited by Dorfman W, Cristofar L. New York, Macmillan, 1985, pp 52–60

Young SJ, Aipers DH, Norland CC: Psychiatric illness and the irritable bowel syndrome. Gastroenterology 70:162–166, 1976

Zisook S, DeVaul RA: Emotional factors in inflammatory bowel disease. South Med J 70:716–719, 1977

CHAPTER 7

Dermatologic Conditions

DAVID G. FOLKS, M.D.

F. CLEVELAND KINNEY, M.D., PH.D.

A survey of the literature reveals few systematic studies of the psychiatry of dermatologic disorders (Van Moffaert 1982). Diseases of the skin significantly affect tactile communication, bodily relationships, and, in particular, sexual contact. Self-inflicted syndromes show a close affinity for and special predilection to the skin. Dermatoses and bodily defects presumably have an enormous impact on an individual's psychosocial functioning. Also, the easy accessibility of the skin enables direct interaction with lesions. Thus, touching, scratching, or exaggeration of lesions; neglecting necessary skin care; or manifest noncompliance with therapeutic regimens may all complicate or result in dermatologic lesions.

Doran and colleagues (1985) summarized dermatologic disturbances with respect to psychological factors that may precipitate, aggravate, or perpetuate disturbances of the skin (Table 7–1). There are also many nonspecific dermatologic conditions that require consideration of psychological factors that may be present and significant—that is, manifest symptoms, personality features, coping styles, stress reactions, and lifestyle factors that affect the dermatologic condition or compliance with medical regimen.

Controlled studies, discussed later, have consistently shown that psychosocial stressors, interpersonal maladjustment, self-esteem, and social stigma are common psychological issues among populations with dermatologic conditions. Psychiatric consultation or assessment, as well as the judicious use of psychotherapy, behavioral techniques, and psychodynamic approaches, is frequently necessary in the clinical management of these patients. Psychotropic medications are frequently prescribed for dermatologic patients; antihistamines, antidepressants, anxiolytics, and lithium compounds have a special role in the pharmacological treatment of dermatologic conditions.

Rationale and Methods

Reports on psychological factors affecting dermatologic conditions in the past decade have substantially strengthened many older concepts regarding the following: 1) the association of stress, 2) the impact of mood and anxiety disorders, 3) the influence and relative importance of social support (or lack thereof), and 4) the role of specific psychological or personality factors (e.g., hostility, perfectionism, low self-esteem) (Ramsay and O'Reagan 1988). Psychobiological studies have just begun to explore psychodermatology with respect to the psychophysiological influences of histamines, prostaglandins, serotonin, norepinephrine, dopamine, and inherent neuroendocrine and immunological mechanisms. Refinements in the study of psychopharmacological agents and the availability of more selective agents have begun to improve our understanding of basic neurobiological mechanisms for these compounds in the treatment of dermatologic conditions. Thus, psychodermatology represents a viable psychosomatic domain for future investigation.

Only those articles that describe rigorous research design and review

TABLE 7–1.   Dermatologic conditions precipitated, aggravated, or perpetuated by psychological factors

Dermatologic condition	Specific examples
Psychogenic disturbance and dermatosis	Neurodermatosis
Hypersensitivity reactions	Pruritus, eczema, urticaria
Stress-induced dermatosis	Shingles, herpes zoster
Metabolic or drug-induced dermatosis	Lithium-induced psoriasis
Neurotic dermatosis	Trichotillomania
Body image disturbances	Acne, seborrhea, psoriasis

Note.   Modified from Doran et al. 1985.

methods or those that report clinical cases in great detail were incorporated in the materials reviewed by the DSM-IV (American Psychiatric Association 1994) Work Group examining psychological factors affecting dermatologic conditions. The outcome of this literature review culminated in a number of significant findings about dermatologic illness and the role of psychological factors (see Table 7–2). However, pruritus, hyperhidrosis, urticaria, acne, atopic dermatitis, and other disease-specific syndromes were not uniformly represented in the literature. A number of reviews and clinical case reports repeatedly addressed the problem of self-induced dermatoses (Doran et al. 1985). The specific dermatologic illnesses of psoriasis (Gupta et al. 1989), chronic urticaria

TABLE 7–2. Psychodermatologic disturbances

Syndrome	Psychological or biobehavioral factors	Conventional clinical treatment
Pruritus	Stress Histamine, prostaglandin E, and endopeptidase mediated	Antihistamine therapy Topical preparations Psychotherapy Anxiolytics
Hyperhydrosis	Stress Excessive eccrine function	Psychotherapy Psychotropics
Atopic dermatitis (eczema)	Stress Familial/developmental factors	Topical preparations Psychotherapy Anxiolytics
Urticaria	Allergic factors (acute) Psychosomatic factors (chronic)	Topical preparations Psychotropics Psychotherapy Antihistamines Systemic steroids
Rosacea	Environmental factors	Psychotropics Stress management Environmental manipulation
Alopecia	Unknown	Stress management Psychotherapy
Psoriasis	Stress Sequelae of infection Environmental factors Drug reaction (especially lithium)	Topical preparations Environmental preparations Psychotherapy Anxiolytics

(Fava et al. 1980), and atopic dermatitis (Faulstich and Williamson 1985) were more frequently the subject of specific inquiry and are the focus of the discussion that follows. The review also identified a number of references analyzing psychotropic agents and dermatologic patients that are discussed later in this chapter.

Disease-Specific Syndromes

Psoriasis

Psoriasis is a chronic, intractable, hyperproliferative skin disease characterized by coalescing erythematous dry patches covered by abundant grayish-white scales. The prevalence in the general population varies geographically from 1% to 2.8% and is estimated to affect 1–3 million people in the United States; the United States prevalence rate is from 0.5% to 1.5%. Approximately 30% of monozygotic twin pairs are concordant for psoriasis (Gupta et al. 1987a). Environmental and genetic factors lead to this disorder. In 60% of the cases, psoriasis starts before the age of 30. The psychological aspects of this disorder are largely associated with the visibility of the disorder and the need for consistent care.

Ginsburg and Link (1989) examined stigmatization issues observed in psoriasis patients. The authors assessed the manner in which 100 adults experienced their illness, as reported on the following six psychological dimensions: 1) anticipation of rejection, 2) feelings of being flawed, 3) sensitivity to other's attitudes, 4) guilt and shame, 5) secretiveness, and 6) positive attitudes. The presence of bleeding psoriatic lesions proved to be the strongest predictor of stigma. Clinical investigators have previously observed how despair and stigmatization result in noncompliance with treatment (Gupta et al. 1989). In another study of stigma, Ramsay and O'Reagan (1988) observed 104 psoriasis patients and found that "social and emotional morbidity" adversely influenced patients' treatment outcome despite easy access to treatment. In fact, 55% of the patients never experienced a complete remission from their psoriasis, which in turn contributed to their avoidance of common social activities (e.g., swimming, the pursuit of sexual relationships). Psoriasis has been associated with depression and case reports of completed suicide. Gupta and colleagues (1993) reported a significant association between depression and suicide ($P < .0001$) in 217 psoriasis patients completing the Carroll Rating Scale for Depression. Moreover, psoriasis severity as perceived by the patient correlated directly with the overall depression scores ($r = .39, P < .0001$).

Gupta and colleagues (Faulstich et al. 1985; Gupta et al. 1989) also examined a subgroup of psoriasis patients depicted as "high stress reactors" who represented a more severely ill subgroup. A strong relationship was shown between patients' perceived psychosocial stress and exacerbations of psoriasis, a finding consistent with similar studies by Payne and colleagues (1985). However, a cause-effect relationship was not clearly shown. Moreover, several authors have noted the profound influence of pruritus on the course of psoriasis (Faulstich et al. 1985; Gaston et al. 1987; Ginsburg and Link 1989; Gupta et al. 1988, 1989; Seville 1977). Prospective study of pertinent psychiatric and dermatologic correlates among 82 inpatients with psoriasis showed that 67% of the cases met clinical criteria for moderate to severe pruritus (Gupta et al. 1988). However, as was the case in the study by Payne and colleagues, pruritus severity did not correlate significantly in the study by Gupta and colleagues (Faulstich et al. 1985; Gupta et al. 1989) with stress associated with life events, age at onset of illness, age, gender, marital status, or average reported daily alcohol consumption. A number of prospective studies of psoriasis and stress have alluded to the difficulty of conducting these investigations (Gaston et al. 1987; Seville 1977). Refinements in diagnosis and research design undoubtedly are necessary if further studies are to address the influence of psychological factors on psoriasis and the prognostic significance of pruritus and other biopsychosocial factors.

Dermatitis

The association between psychological factors and the various general dermatoses (e.g., eczematous, atopic, and pruritic dermatitis) has not been systematically investigated. Anxiety and mood disorders and specific psychophysiological syndromes, such as migraine headache and irritable bowel syndrome, have been frequently reported to coexist in cases of dermatoses (Garvey and Tollefson 1988); specifically, the role of abnormal serotonergic mechanisms has been implicated (Garvey and Tollefson 1988). In one study that controlled for sociodemographics and medical status, stress in the family environment was found to predict a patient's severity of symptoms (Gil et al. 1987). Faulstich and colleagues (Faulstich and Williamson 1985; Faulstich et al. 1985) systematically evaluated 10 atopic dermatitis patients with active symptomatology and compared these cases with 10 control subjects matched for age, gender, and race. Both groups were given a stressful set of tasks to complete. Compared with control subjects, the 10 atopic dermatitis patients showed greater electromyogram and heart rate activity and higher anxiety scores on the Symptom Checklist—90-Revised. A similar study by Fjellner and Arnetz (1985) evaluated psychological predictors of pruritus during mental stress, and they also concluded that dermatosis characterized by pruritus may be exacerbated by emotional stress. During the control period, the subjects under study listened to relaxation tapes and thereafter were exposed to mental stressors for 50 minutes, followed by another 40-minute recovery phase. The results of this study confirmed that pruritus was significantly influenced by psychological stress. This study showed that interindividual differences among patients and control subjects were pronounced; Fjellner and Arnetz hypothesized that the observed differences in urinary adrenaline response pattern were an important correlate to manifest symptoms (i.e., adrenaline appeared to have a suppressive effect on itch and an enhanced effect on flare responses), and pulse rate was shown to correlate positively with flare.

The psychobiological influences affecting pruritic dermatosis range from a low-grade sensation to a painful experience that often benefits from pharmacotherapy (e.g., antihistamines, antidepressants). A review of well-established pharmacological treatments is beyond the scope of this review; the reader is referred elsewhere (Folks and Kinney 1991). The current literature suggests that skin testing and allergy consultation are often indicated and should include eosinophil counts, sedimentation rate, and other appropriate laboratory screening that might aid the clinician in determining allergic responses or parasitic infestation (e.g., scabies, lice). Reports of eosinophilia myalgia associated with tryptophan illustrate the need to consider carefully the possible etiologic role of drugs and food (Clauw et al. 1990).

Acne

The relationship between psychological factors and acne is commonly inferred. Acne patients report a high frequency of diminished self-esteem and often show negative self-image (Rubinow et al. 1987). Anxiety-depression, psychological symptoms arising from low self-esteem, and subsequent social withdrawal are known clinical concomitants of more severe forms of acne. Van der Meeren and colleagues (1985) followed a group of 40 patients with severe acne and examined their personality factors and clinical course; "neuroticism," "social extraversion," and "self-defensive attitude" were identified as the more adaptive subtypes. This subgroup reportedly displayed lower self-defensive attitudes than did control subjects. A subgroup of 12 patients with conglobate acne were successfully treated with isotretinoin and were reevaluated after 1 year using a core psychometric battery. Personality factors had not consistently changed among the more severely affected individuals. However, symptoms of anxiety-depression were found to be significantly diminished after successful treatment outcome. Wu and colleagues (1988) also examined the possible role of personality and emotional factors in acne patients. As with the findings of Van der Meeren and colleagues, emotional disturbances involving symptoms of anxiety and anger were found as the only significant psychological factors.

Other systematic studies of acne patients that evaluate various psychiatric factors in response to treatment using isotretinoin, local treatment, or antibiotics have not been adequately addressed in the literature (Folks and Kinney 1991). Psychotherapeutic approaches to patients with severe acne who manifest adjustment disorders certainly deserve further study, specifically of the efficacy or impact of psychological or psychiatric interventions on a patient's course. Disfiguring acne with subsequent disturbances of body image presumably would require comprehensive approaches using supportive psychotherapy or perhaps other sophisticated psychological techniques. However, systematic studies have not provided data or rationale supporting this general treatment approach.

Urticaria

In the United States, 15%–20% of the population is afflicted with urticaria on at least one occasion (Monroe 1988). Urticaria or "hives" refers to a typical skin reaction that is classically described as the wheal and flare response and is arbitrarily considered chronic when it has persisted for more than 12 weeks. The accepted theory of the mechanism for cutaneous anaphylaxis or hive formation is similar to that explaining the pathogenesis of systemic anaphylaxis (Sell 1990). The etiologic factors implicated in the development of chronic urticaria are difficult to determine. A review of 236 cases by Shertzer and Lookingbill (1987) concluded that psychological factors are frequently implicated or judged etiologic. Of course, the relationship between stress and urticaria has been generally accepted, but future studies need to consider carefully whether specific psychophysiological and psychosocial factors are definitively associated. Without doubt, drugs may precipitate the formation of urticaria; both parenteral and oral ingestion are implicated in acute urticarial reactions. Conventional wisdom admonishes clinicians to discontinue a specific pharmaceutical agent that is potentially implicated in an acute urticarial reaction, regardless of severity. Traditionally, antihistamines are used in the treatment of both acute and chronic urticaria, including the recent use of terfenadine, an H_1 antagonist that does not exhibit the prominent anticholinergic side effects attributed to other antihistaminic compounds. The tricyclic antidepressant doxepin (in doses of 30–75 mg) and other tricyclic agents with similar effects (i.e., competitive blockers of both H_1 and H_2 receptors) are widely used by dermatologists for the treatment of chronic urticaria (Greene et al. 1985; Neittaanmaki and Fraki 1988). Although antihistaminic agents do not cure urticaria, they do serve to control the overt manifestations. Interestingly, systemic steroids are rarely useful in the treatment of urticaria.

Self-Induced Dermatoses

Factitious dermatoses have been recognized since 1863, when Gavin first reported a case of factitious scabies in a sailor who rubbed gun powder into needle punctures on his wrist. The incidence of dermatitis artefacta, or factitial dermatitis (Folks et al. 1994), is 0.3% among dermatologic patients and is observed predominantly among females; the age at onset reportedly spans a broad range of 9–73 years. A comprehensive review, beyond the scope of this chapter, is provided elsewhere (Doran et al. 1985; Folks et al. 1994).

Essentially, lesions resulting from factitial dermatosis have wide-ranging morphologic features and are often bizarre looking with sharp geometric borders surrounded by normal-looking skin. More serious lesions can result in complications, such as infection (Earle and Folks 1986), or in the escalation of symptoms in the case of factitial behavior (Folks and Houck 1993). Self-inflicted dermatologic lesions frequently have been associated with mental retardation, psychosis, factitious disorders including Munchausen's syndrome, and malingering. Focusing on factitial dermatologic conditions, Folks and Freeman (1985) outlined the management principles most likely to result in a successful therapy (Table 7–3). Psychiatric consultation and psychological testing, such as Amytal interview or hypnosis, may also improve clinical management. Gupta and colleagues (1987b) addressed the self-inflicted dermatoses and differentiated dermatitis artefacta, neurotic excoriations, and trichotillomania. They then eloquently depicted specific associations between these three entities and their various degrees of psychopathology. However, these three related diagnostic categories of self-destructive dermatoses have received little emphasis in the psychiatric literature; in fact, only case reports or clinical reviews are prominent. Gupta and colleagues, like Folks and Freeman, emphasized the need for identifying any underlying disorders (e.g., anxiety, depression, psychotic disturbance)

TABLE 7–3. Aspects of Munchausen's syndrome and other factitious illnesses potentially amenable to treatment

- Psychiatric syndromes
  Affective disorders
  Anxiety disorders
  Psychotic disorders
  Conversion disorders
  Substance abuse disorders
  Organic mental disorders
- Personality organization closer to compulsive, depressive, or histrionic rather than borderline, narcissistic, or antisocial

- Stability in psychosocial support system as manifested by marriage, stable occupation, family ties as opposed to the single, unemployed wanderer
- Ability to cope with confrontation or some redefinition of the illness behavior
- Capability of establishing and maintaining rapport with the treating clinicians

Source. Modified from Folks and Freeman 1985.

that are more readily amenable to intervention. The methodology of Colon and colleagues (1991) utilized the Diagnostic Interview Schedule among a dermatologic group with alopecia areata. A significant percentage of psychiatric disturbance (74%) was found. Major depression (39%) and generalized anxiety (39%) were noteworthy lifetime prevalence rates. This study calls attention to the need for psychiatric assessment in other dermatologic populations.

Dermatologic Conditions and the Role of Psychotropic Medications

Psychotropics prescribed for individuals who develop or display dermatologic disorders include a broad spectrum of pharmacological agents, including antipsychotics, antidepressants, anxiolytics, and various miscellaneous compounds. The role of these drugs with respect to the dermatologic condition, directly or indirectly, continues to be clarified in the literature. Psychotropic drugs, especially lithium and the antidepressants, are frequently associated with adverse dermatologic reactions. The literature discussed below affirms the importance of the drug-disease relationship and the ongoing need to study these agents with respect to the diagnostic and therapeutic approach to dermatologic conditions.

Neuroleptics

Chlorpromazine-induced discoloration of skin exposed to sunlight was first described in 1964 by Greiner and Berry. Lovell and colleagues (1986) reported an interesting case in which photocontact urticaria developed, also presumably due to chlorpromazine. Thus, a novel and consequential dermatologic effect in contrast to delayed, photosensitive eczema is now under consideration (i.e., an urticarial reaction that is *not* due to an alteration in the molecular structure of the drug as an allergen, but rather as an in vivo drug effect). Similarly, positive photopatch testing and recurrence of generalized maculopapular eruption following allergy testing has been identified with thioridazine treatment at doses of 60 mg daily (Thompson et al. 1988). The precise mechanism for the adverse skin reactions reported in this latter case also represents a viable topic for future study. With regard to the nonphenothiazine agents, a detailed case report noted the disappearance of the abnormal skin pigmentation that had been associated with phenothiazine treatment when haloperidol was instituted (Ban et al. 1985). Similarly, Thompson and colleagues reported four chronic psychiatric patients who received prolonged high-dose chlorpromazine therapy when cutaneous pigmentation resolved after haloperidol was substituted. However, in these four cases, chlorpromazine-induced corneal and lenticular opacities persisted. An international study by Ban and colleagues (1985) repudiated the claims that haloperidol is without potential for skin reactions or that it can actually reverse the adverse effects of phenothiazines. Current data suggest that any neuroleptic should be regarded as potentially inducing an idiosyncratic or allergic reaction, even though more potent neuroleptics continue to be reported as less dermatoxic (e.g., pimozide, haloperidol, thiothixene, fluphenazine) (Folks and Kinney 1991).

Psychotropic-Intrinsic Allergens

Tartrazine (FD&C Yellow No. 5) and other dye sensitivities have been implicated in the etiology of skin reactions. Pohl and colleagues (1987) described five cases of apparent allergy to tartrazine in 170 exposed patients. This frequency of 6/1,000 was higher than that previously reported. As a consequence, tartrazine has been removed from two psychotropic drugs: imipramine and desipramine. Urticarial bronchospasms and nonthrombocytopenic papular rashes have also been anecdotally associated with tartrazine, and it is conceivable that angioedema, rhinitis, and anaphylaxis might also be precipitated by tartrazine (T. Barnard, Sandoz Pharmaceuticals, East Hanover, NJ, personal communication, November 1988). Reports of allergic reactions to lithium compounds including anaphylaxis and delayed-type hypersensitivity are also now well documented (Clark and Jefferson 1987; Lockey 1959). The possibility remains that the drug reactions associated with lithium and other agents are due in part or primarily to inert ingredients.

Antidepressants

Cutaneous reactions to antidepressants may include acneform eruptions, seborrheic dermatitis, contact dermatitis, nonspecific pruritic eruptions, and urticarial or photosensitivity reactions (Folks and Kinney 1991). These acute dermatologic conditions are generally benign and self-limited. Transient photosensitivity reactions have also been reported with tricyclic antidepressants and structurally related compounds. Walter-Ryan and colleagues (1985) reported a case of a previously healthy 38-year-old patient with anxiety-depression who developed a reversible rash after treatment with imipramine. Resolution of the rash after discontinuation of imipramine and a subsequent challenge with maprotiline was uneventful. Tricyclic-induced photosensitivity reactions similar to this case report are postulated to occur in the following situations: 1) when the parent drug produces phytotoxicity or photoallergy, 2) when drug photosensitivity products produced in the skin by ultraviolet light become toxic, or 3) when fixed drug eruptions occur as the drug or its metabolites form complexes with nucleic acids and are bound in the skin. These three mechanisms are presumptive but congruent with the cutaneous reactions known to be associated with chlorpromazine and protriptyline (Walter-Ryan et al. 1985). Oral ingestion of the antidepressant fluoxetine hydrochloride may result in dermatologic side effects infrequently observed as acne, alopecia, contact dermatitis, dry skin, herpes simplex, maculopapular rash, and urticaria (D. Wheadon, Dista Pharmaceuticals, Indianapolis, IN, personal communication, November 1988). These dermatologic complications, more rarely observed with fluoxetine, are presumably allergic reactions that have been observed and reported in placebo-controlled clinical trials (Wheadon, personal communication).

Erythema multiforme is an acute, usually self-limited syndrome that produces distinctive skin lesions both with and without mucosal erosions. The classic mild form described in the mid-1800s can, however, progress to a more severe and sometimes fatal form that was first described by Stevens and Johnson (1922). Ford and Jenike (1985) reported a case of a 63-year-old woman with depression who was treated with trazodone and her subsequent development of erythema multiforme. Interestingly, the patient in this case was also taking lithium, which had not been previously implicated in the development of erythema multiforme.

Although many of the previously mentioned adverse reactions can result from antidepressant medication, many antidepressant agents are also effective in the treatment of certain dermatologic conditions, such as neurodermatitis and chronic urticaria (Greene et al. 1985). Eedy and Corbett (1987) described a patient who presented with facial hyperhidrosis characterized by a bilateral malar distribution precipitated by olfactory stimuli who was successfully treated with amitriptyline. Similarly, Yeragani and colleagues (1988) reported a case of a 30-year-old male with major depression and coexisting skin disease diagnosed as dyshidrosis. This patient had 1- to 2-mm papules on the palmar surfaces of both hands that had been continuously present for about 2.5 years. Desipramine treatment, at a blood level of 150 ng/ml, resulted in marked improvement in the patient's skin condition. Because the therapeutic effect was not likely to have been caused by any antihistaminic effect of desipramine or from an anticholinergic effect, the therapeutic mechanism of action proposed was a decreased autonomic instability that resulted in a decrease in stress-induced dermatologic symptoms. This case illustrates the need to consider conventional antidepressant agents and their effectiveness in dermatoses in which a therapeutic response results from restoring autonomic and homeostatic mechanisms, especially during periods of psychological stress.

Lithium

Gupta and colleagues (1986) provided an excellent review of psychotropic drugs and dermatology focusing on lithium compounds. In the lithium-psoriasis association, lithium increases both circulating and marginal polymorphonuclear leukocyte pools and in turn enhances their turnover and migration. Concurrently, lithium inhibits the enzyme adenylate cyclase, thereby lowering levels of adenosine 3',5'-cyclic monophosphate (cAMP) and enhancing neutrophil chemotaxis (Heng 1982; Jefferson et al. 1983; Lazarus and Gilgor 1979). These changes purportedly result in epidermal cell proliferation that leads to a nonpustular form of psoriasis and a diverse spectrum of dermatologic side effects (Alvarez and Freinhar 1984).

Although psoriasis is known to be exacerbated by lithium, alopecia (hair loss) is not commonly observed in association with lithium. Mortimer and Dawber (1984) reviewed and commented on the association between lithium and alopecia, as did Ghadirian and Lalinec-Michaud (1986) and Vacaflor and colleagues (1970), who reported a lithium-induced alopecia that reversed with the discontinuation of the drug. Mortimer and Dawber concluded that alopecia does indeed result from lithium therapy per se, but they also noted that patients usually recover despite continuation of lithium treatment. Silvestri and colleagues (1988) reported a case where global alopecia was observed during lithium therapy followed by improvement with the suspension of lithium therapy.

Sarantidis and Waters (1983) noted the incidence of a variety of cutaneous conditions among 91 lithium-treated patients compared with 44 patients treated with other nonneuroleptic psychotropics. Structured interviews, demographics, medication histories, and personal and family histories were obtained in this study. A significantly greater proportion of the lithium-treated patients showed a cutaneous condition secondary to drug treatment that was either an initial onset or an exacerbation of a preexisting condition; 28 patients developed psoriasis, 17 developed acne, 12 developed folliculitis, and 7 developed a maculopapular rash. Clark and Jefferson (1987) described a case in which lithium exacerbated a preexisting, biopsy-confirmed Darier's disease (keratosis follicularis) with subsequent improvement on discontinuation. A recurrence, or exacerbation, after a secondary exposure to lithium was also observed in this case. The mechanism of this response was proposed to be similar to lithium and psoriasis (i.e., the inhibition of cAMP and subsequent in vivo increase in the proliferation of epidermal cells).

Discussion and Recommendations

A diagnostic and nosologic schema is needed that would better link psychological factors and dermatologic conditions. Moreover, pharmacological influences affecting the cause, course, or outcome of dermatologic disorders deserve specific inquiry that uses rigorous research design. The current data base is largely descriptive and presumptive at best, with the exception of the well-established relationship between lithium compounds and psoriasis.

A nosologic format that systematically addresses the role of psychological and psychiatric factors is the logical next step in the biopsychosocial approach to dermatologic conditions. Dermatologic conditions and their association with psychological or biobehavioral factors contain many potential areas of inquiry, including the following: 1) stress response syndromes; 2) mood disorders (e.g., anxiety-depression); 3) psychosocial factors (e.g., family constellation, coping styles, interpersonal relationships); 4) psychobiological factors (e.g., histamines, prostaglandins, serotonin, norepinephrine, dopamine, psychoimmunology); and 5) continued assessment of personality factors (i.e., hostility or perfectionism and psychological concomitants of self-esteem).

The role of psychological factors in dermatologic conditions and clarification of the therapeutic and nontherapeutic effects of the psychotropics is an area of psychosomatic medicine that could benefit greatly from an improved diagnostic approach (Stoudemire and Hales 1991). A nosologic advance may also allow clinicians to appreciate and address treatment strategies better and improve clinical management significantly. In addition to prospective designs and longitudinal studies, a diagnostic system that specifies the nature of psychological or behavioral factors as proposed for the revision of the DSM-III-R (American Psychiatric Association 1987) category of "psychological factors affecting physical conditions" may improve the quality and depth of future investigations.

References

Alvarez WA, Freinhar JP: Direct evidence for a lithium-induced psoriasis syndrome. Int J Psychosom 31:21–22, 1984

American Psychiatric Association: Diagnostic and Statistical Manual of Mental Disorders, 3rd Edition, Revised. Washington, DC, American Psychiatric Association, 1987

American Psychiatric Association: Diagnostic and Statistical Manual of Mental Disorders, 4th Edition. Washington, DC, American Psychiatric Association, 1994

Ban TA, Guy W, Wilson WH: Neuroleptic-induced skin pigmentation in chronic hospitalized schizophrenic patients. Can J Psychiatry 30:406–408, 1985

Clark KJ, Jefferson JW: Lithium allergy (letter). J Clin Psychopharmacol 7:287–289, 1987

Clauw DJ, Nashel DJ, Umhau A, et al: Tryptophan-associated eosinophilic connective-tissue disease. JAMA 263:1502–1506, 1990

Colon EA, Popkin MK, Callies AL, et al: Lifetime prevalence of psychiatric disorders in patients with alopecia areata. Compr Psychiatry 32:245–251, 1991

Doran AR, Roy A, Wolkowitz OM: Self-destructive dermatoses. Psychiatr Clin North Am 8:291–298, 1985

Earle JR, Folks DG: Factitious disorder and coexisting depression: a report of successful psychiatric consultation and case management. Gen Hosp Psychiatry 8:448–450, 1986

Eedy DJ, Corbett JR: Olfactory facial hyperhydrosis responding to amitriptyline. Clin Exp Dermatol 12:298–299, 1987

Faulstich ME, Williamson DA: An overview of atopic dermatitis: toward a biobehavioral integration. J Psychosom Res 29:647–654, 1985

Faulstich ME, Williamson DA, Duchmann EG, et al: Psychophysiological analysis of atopic dermatitis. J Psychosom Res 29:415–417, 1985

Fava GA, Perini GI, Santonastaso P, et al: Life events and psychological distress in dermatologic disorders: psoriasis, chronic urticaria, and fungal infections. Br J Med Psychol 53:277–282, 1980

Fjellner B, Arnetz BB: Psychological predictors of pruritus during mental stress. Acta Derm Venereol (Stockh) 65:504–508, 1985

Folks DG, Freeman AM: Munchausen's syndrome and other factitious illness. Psychiatr Clin North Am 8:263–278, 1985

Folks DG, Houck C: Somatoform disorders, factitious disorders, and malingering, in Psychiatric Care of the Medical Patient. Edited by Stoudemire A, Fogel BS. New York, Oxford University Press, 1993, pp 267–287

Folks DG, Kinney FC: Dermatology, in Medical Psychiatric Practice. Edited by Stoudemire A, Fogel BS. Washington, DC, American Psychiatric Press, 1991, pp 287–308

Folks DG, Ford CV, Houck CA: Somatoform disorders, factitious disorders, and malingering, in Clinical Psychiatry for Medical Students, 2nd Edition. Edited by Stoudemire A. Philadelphia, PA, JB Lippincott, 1994, pp 274–305

Ford HE, Jenike MA: Erythema multiform associated with trazodone therapy: case report. J Clin Psychiatry 46:294–295, 1985

Garvey MJ, Tollefson GD: Association of affective disorder with migraine headaches and neurodermatitis. Gen Hosp Psychiatry 10:148–149, 1988

Gaston L, Lassonde M, Bernier-Buzzanga J, et al: Psoriasis and stress: a prospective study. J Am Acad Dermatol 17:82–86, 1987

Gavin H: Feigned and Fictitious Diseases, Chiefly of Soldiers and Seamen. London, Churchill, 1863

Ghadirian AM, Lalinec-Michaud M: Report of a patient with lithium-related alopecia and psoriasis. J Clin Psychiatry 47:212–213, 1986

Gil KM, Keefe FJ, Sampson HA, et al: The relation of stress and family environment to atopic dermatitis symptoms in children. J Psychosom Res 31:673–684, 1987

Ginsburg IH, Link BG: Feelings of stigmatization in patients with psoriasis. J Am Acad Dermatol 20:53–63, 1989

Greene SL, Reed CE, Schroeter AL: Double-blind crossover study comparing doxepin with diphenhydramine for the treatment of chronic urticaria. J Am Acad Dermatol 12:669–675, 1985

Greiner AC, Berry K: Skin pigmentation and corneal and lens opacities with prolonged chlorpromazine therapy. Can Med Assoc J 90:663–665, 1964

Gupta MA, Gupta AK, Haberman HF: Psychotropic drugs in dermatology. J Am Acad Dermatol 14:633–645, 1986

Gupta MA, Gupta AK, Haberman HF: Psoriasis and psychiatry: an update. Gen Hosp Psychiatry 9:157–166, 1987a

Gupta MA, Gupta AK, Haberman HF: The self-inflicted dermatoses: a critical review. Gen Hosp Psychiatry 9:45–52, 1987b

Gupta MA, Gupta AK, Kirkby S, et al: Pruritus in psoriasis: a prospective study of some psychiatric and dermatologic correlates. Arch Dermatol 124:1052–1057, 1988

Gupta MA, Gupta AK, Kirkby S, et al: A psychocutaneous profile of psoriasis patients who are stress reactors. Gen Hosp Psychiatry 11:166–173, 1989

Gupta MA, Schork NJ, Gupta AK, et al: Suicidal ideation in psoriasis. Int J Dermatol 32:188–190, 1993

Heng MCY: Cutaneous manifestations of lithium toxicity. Br J Dermatol 106:107–109, 1982

Jefferson JW, Griest JH, Ackerman DL: Lithium Encyclopedia for Clinical Practice. Washington, DC, American Psychiatric Press, 1983

Lazarus GS, Gilgor RS: Psoriasis, polymorphonuclear leukocytes, and lithium carbonate: important clue. Arch Dermatol 115:1183–1184, 1979

Lockey SD: Allergic reactions due to FD and C Yellow No. 5 tartrazine, an aniline dye used as a coloring and identifying agent in various steroids. Ann Allergy 17:719–721, 1959

Lovell CR, Cronin E, Rhodes EL: Photocontact urticaria from chlorpromazine. Contact Dermatitis 14:290–291, 1986

Monroe EW: Urticaria, in Common Problems in Dermatology. Edited by Green KE. Chicago, IL, Year Book Medicine, 1988, pp 402–407

Mortimer PS, Dawber RPR: Hair loss and lithium. Int J Dermatol 23:603–604, 1984

Neittaanmaki H, Fraki JE: Combination of localized heat urticaria and cold urticaria: release of histamine in suction blisters and successful treatment of heat urticaria with doxepin. Clin Exp Dermatol 13:87–91, 1988

Payne RA, Payne CME, Marks R: Stress does not worsen psoriasis?—a controlled study of 32 patients. Clin Exp Dermatol 10:239–245, 1985

Pohl R, Balon R, Berchou R, et al: Allergy to tartrazine in antidepressants. Am J Psychiatry 144:237–238, 1987

Ramsay B, O'Reagan M: A survey of the social and psychological effects of psoriasis. Br J Dermatol 118:195–201, 1988

Rubinow DR, Peck GL, Squillace KM, et al: Reduced anxiety and depression in cystic acne patients after successful treatment with oral isotretinoin. J Am Acad Dermatol 17:25–32, 1987

Sarantidis D, Waters B: A review and controlled study of cutaneous conditions associated with lithium carbonate. Br J Psychiatry 143:42–50, 1983

Sell S: Immunopathology (hypersensitivity diseases), in Anderson's Pathology, 9th Edition. Edited by Kissane JE. St. Louis, MO, CV Mosby, 1990, pp 487–545

Seville RH: Psoriasis and stress. Br J Dermatol 97:297–302, 1977

Shertzer CL, Lookingbill DP: Effects of relaxation therapy and hypnotizability in chronic urticaria. Arch Dermatol 123:913–916, 1987

Silvestri A, Santonastaso P, Paggiarin D: Alopecia areata during lithium therapy: a case report. Gen Hosp Psychiatry 10:46–48, 1988

Stevens AM, Johnson FC: A new eruptive fever associated with stomatitis and ophthalmia. Am J Dis Child 24:526–533, 1922

Stoudemire A, Hales RE: Psychological and behavioral factors affecting medical conditions and DSM-IV: an overview. Psychosomatics 32:5–13, 1991

Thompson TR, Lai S, Yassa R, et al: Resolution of chlorpromazine-induced pigmentation with haloperidol substitution. Acta Psychiatr Scand 78:763–765, 1988

Vacaflor L, Lehmann HE, Ban TA: Side effects and teratogenicity of lithium carbonate treatment. J Clin Pharmacol 10:387, 1970

Van der Meeren HLM, Van der Schaar WW, Van den Hurk CMAM: The psychological impact of severe acne. Cutis 36:84–86, 1985

Van Moffaert M: Psychosomatics for the practicing dermatologist. Dermatologica 165:73–87, 1982

Walter-Ryan WG, Kern EE, Shiriff JR, et al: Persistent photoaggravated cutaneous eruption induced by imipramine (letter). JAMA 254:357–358, 1985

Wu SF, Kinder BN, Trunnell TN, et al: Role of anxiety and anger in acne patients: a relationship with the severity of the disorder. J Am Acad Dermatol 18:325–333, 1988

Yeragani VK, Patel H, Keshavan MS: Effectiveness of desipramine in the treatment of dyshydrosis (letter). J Clin Psychopharmacol 8:76–77, 1988

CHAPTER 8

Pulmonary and Rheumatologic Diseases

MICHAEL G. MORAN, M.D.

There is a great deal of anecdotal information regarding the effects of psychological factors (variously called "stress," "depression," and "psychosocial stressors") on pulmonary and rheumatologic illnesses. Most of the research in this area has been conducted on two illnesses that are representative of the two categories and the respective research problems for the two disease groups: asthma and rheumatoid arthritis. These two diseases are used as the focus for this chapter. A major conclusion that is drawn from this review is that most studies that now exist—retrospective and inconsistent in design, patient selection, and nomenclature—provide an inadequate basis for reliable inferences about the associations between psychological factors and pulmonary and rheumatologic disease. This comment is not seen as an argument against the usefulness of the DSM-IV (American Psychiatric Association 1994) category, "psychological factors affecting medical condition," but rather as an indicator of the need for more study.

Pulmonary Disease

Asthma

Asthma has long been considered one of the "psychosomatic" diseases by both patients and physicians. In ascribing asthma this notoriety, it has been implied that both patients and physicians have seen or experienced at least an association between patients' psychological and pulmonary functioning. From the 1930s through the 1950s, asthma was a charter member of the pantheon of the "holy seven" psychosomatic illnesses (Dunbar 1947). Psychoanalytic theories of the time purported to describe the etiology of asthma as psychological (Alexander 1950) and even went so far as to suggest that the critical and specific psychosomatic dilemma was one of conflicted unconscious dependency wishes (French and Alexander 1941). These summary notions had been formulated from analyses of adult asthmatic patients via the reconstruction of childhood traumatic events. The pathogenic chain was then hypothesized in the following causal sequence: childhood trauma leads to unconscious conflict over dependency, which leads to unacceptability of direct expression of conflict, which leads to somatic manifestation of conflict (asthma). Even though systematic studies were lacking, hypotheses of this sort gained considerable vogue. One point that should not be lost: the notions had beginnings in patient and physician experience.

Many patients were treated for asthma and for a number of other conditions that were considered psychogenic in origin (or sensitive to influence through psychogenic mechanisms) by analysis or other talking cures. The treatment of depression was considered especially important for asthmatic patients; psychoanalysts (and nonpsychiatric physicians) came to see the wheeze as the suppressed cry of the child for its mother (French and Alexander 1941). Practitioners of the time also considered other events important in the unconscious life of asthmatic patients, requiring treatment: primal-scene exposure in childhood, sibling birth, mother's miscarriage during pregnancy with a sibling, and death of a close family member (Karol 1980–1981; Teiramaa 1979). The logic of the "choice" of the pulmonary system as the target for the somatic expression of conflict has seldom been pursued, apart from its symbolic usefulness, as in the purported production of a "suppressed cry."

Authors writing in more contemporary times tend to place at least equal emphasis on the physiological mechanisms driving asthma. Some, such as Knapp and Mathe (1985), brought a sophisticated understanding of both the physiological and the psychological to their efforts. A representative causal chain from such a theory might proceed as follows: important psychological events are attributed meaning with correlates in brain-based physiological processes, which in turn result in changes in

autonomic and immunologic activity; these changes in turn effect pathologic pulmonary events through humoral, cell-mediated, and autonomic
pathways. The classic target organ responses then ensue: bronchospasm
(with wheezing on the clinical level), cough, and mucous production.

A brief summary of some of the factors involved in the pathophysiology of an asthma attack facilitates later discussion of this proposed chain
of events. An asthma attack consists, in part, of a state of relative beta$_2$-
adrenergic blockade (Cugell and Fish 1978). For this reason, the use of
beta$_2$-adrenergic blocking drugs, such as propranolol, is relatively con-
traindicated for asthmatic patients. The result might be seen as a relative
dominance of the parasympathetic system's activity, the neurologically
based arm of asthma's pathogenesis. The humoral and cell-mediated arms
are hypothesized as mediated by macrophages, polymorphonuclear cells,
and probably mast cells, in the form of an inflammatory response. Experimental triggering of this arm probably occurs in the instances of those
attacks seen in aspirin-sensitive individuals who take aspirin. Arachido-
nic acid metabolites such as leukotrienes and prostaglandins participate
in this mechanism.

Direct and indirect sympathomimetic agonists are mainstays in the
treatment of most asthmatic episodes and are often used as maintenance
drugs in the absence of overt symptoms. From this clinical fact comes
more support for a "balance" hypothesis (balance between parasympathetic and sympathetic influences) in the etiology and pathophysiology of
asthma.

Thus, a critical research question is as follows: how do emotional
states impinge on these pathophysiological mechanisms? More particularly, perhaps, how do mental phenomena affect the "balance" between
functional parasympathetic and functional sympathetic activity? An in-
terpretive dilemma arises, however; how does the confounding presence
of anxiety as a provocative influence affect the occurrence and exacerbation of asthma attacks? Anxiety should induce a state of relative sympathetic dominance and therefore decrease symptoms rather than *trigger* an
attack. How, therefore, can the demonstration that "stress" and other
emotional disruptions have been causally linked with reductions in airway caliber and with asthma attacks by some researchers be explained
(Bengtsson 1984)? One (at least partial) answer may be found in an intriguing study in which asthmatic patients did not increase secretion of epi-

nephrine during stressful events as much as healthy control subjects (Mathe and Knapp 1969).

On a different hierarchical level, patients and practitioners, as well as some researchers, have attributed increased susceptibility to asthma in the instances of certain personality traits and types. For patients with these traits, risk is deemed higher for asthma or for its most severe manifestations. High-risk personality types include those patients characterized by extreme inhibition, covert aggression, marked dependency needs, high need for affection, and simply "neurosis" (Sharma and Nandkumar 1980). Some workers found that protection from the worst sequelae of asthma was conferred by "extroversion." Depression, anxiety, and disturbances of self-esteem, on the other hand, were considered risk factors (Plutchik et al. 1978). Among asthmatic children, severe psychopathology, psychotic signs, and excessive aggression raises the risk of death due to asthma (Mascia et al. 1989).

Loss or intense disappointment may also increase a patient's susceptibility for asthma attack. Losses in an intense, close, personal relationship have been associated with acute onset of symptoms of asthma. "Early marital life" alone, according to some workers, may increase disease activity (Teiramaa 1981). More broadly, intense "stress" in combination with a limited support system were found in asthmatic patients requiring the highest doses of corticosteroids for symptom control (DeArujo et al. 1973). This finding may be worth exploring further: Do high stress and little support constitute the pathogenic influence? Or is the important—and therefore exacerbating—factor the paucity of practical day-to-day assistance with this illness, with a greater likelihood of resorting to the "big gun" therapy of steroids?

There are few animal studies in this arena. One might account for the paucity of work by the lack of a good animal model for asthma. Two investigatory groups have shown that painful, fear-inducing conditions were likely to induce wheezing (not asthma per se) (Gantt 1944; Schiavi et al. 1951).

The ability to report symptoms can be adversely affected by emotional variables. Thus, through an indirect route can asthma be worsened by psychological factors. For example, personality style may influence a patient's perception of experimentally controlled respiratory pressure load; the more anxious and "dependent" subjects (asthmatic or not) rated the experimentally selected pressure loads higher than did those subjects assessed as having more adaptive styles (Hudgel et al. 1982). Through another, as yet unknown mechanism, sleep loss can reduce an individual's ability to recognize an increase in airway resistance (R. Martin, personal communication, April 1989). This finding may have treatment implications for a variety of conditions associated with sleep disturbances, including major depression.

Both the awareness of and the ability to report affect associated with a loss may also have bearing on the asthmatic patient's condition. A maladaptive response, with inadequate or inappropriate expression of affect, may then be associated with an attack (Knapp 1969; Rees 1956). Alexithymic asthma patients, whose ability to express affect may be compromised, may thus be at risk in the setting of loss. Psychoeducational groups may help and can even be cost effective (Lehrer et al. 1992).

Most investigators working at the junction of somatic and psychological influences on asthma see attacks as multideterminant in etiology. The three most commonly cited precipitants in two reviews were infections, allergens, and emotional stressors (Tunsater 1984; Weiner 1977). The coincident occurrence of precipitants was considered especially likely to induce an episode. Thus, the unitary concept of disease etiology for asthma (either psychological or physiological) is now considered incomplete. For example, researchers understand asthma deaths in children to result from disruptions of a fragile milieu of interdependent components consisting of physiological, pharmacological, and interpersonal factors (Friedman 1984). Another example is reflected in the work of a group at the National Jewish Center in Denver, Colorado, that examined the effects of depression in asthmatic children (Miller and Strunk 1989). Increased mortality seems to be associated with this combination; parasympathetic pathways may be important in the mechanism (B. Miller, personal communication, June 1989).

Chronic Obstructive Pulmonary Disease (COPD)

COPD has been the subject of much less investigation than asthma. Although little has been done in terms of prospective, physiologically based studies, an important body of clinical experience has been reported (Agle and Baum 1977; Clark and Cochrane 1970).

Many surveys of the personality and affective characteristics of COPD patients confirm each other (Weiner 1985). However, these personality "types," once considered common among these patients, have never been carefully excluded as adaptations to a severe chronic illness, as opposed to factors in the etiology or maintenance of COPD.

The symptoms of COPD, such as dyspnea, can vary a great deal, although objective measurements of physiological parameters remain unchanged and within normal limits. Dyspnea "out of proportion" to the pertinent clinical measurements (e.g., of airway resistance) can be augmented or maintained by states of depression, anxiety, or "hysteria" (Burns and Howell 1969). Beyond an effect on the symptom, the functional state of the COPD patient can also suffer during disruptions of mood and motivation. Personality disorders and major disturbances in development contribute to functional disability in these patients (Geddes 1984; Sandhu 1986). On a more behavioral level, conditioning experiences such as breath-holding and crying may play a part in emotional dysregulation and thus worsen dyspnea. Some COPD (and asthma) patients may interpret the dyspnea that can occur during sexual intercourse as the harbinger of a relapse of pulmonary disease. As a result, they may inhibit their intimate involvement with others. This could obviously affect the potential for future relationships or the maintenance of a current one. The adoption of an abnormally and potentially unnecessarily restricted emotional and physical life initiates a vicious cycle of inhibition, decreased functional status, and further emotional and physical inhibition (Dudley et al. 1968). Maladaptive avoidant responses may follow and can include the severe limitation of a wide range of interpersonal activities, as well as the isolation and suppression of intense emotions such as anger (Dudley et al. 1980). The patient may "de-habilitate," and lose stability in cardiovascular conditioning, with an obvious increase in the burden on the primary pulmonary condition (Fishman and Petty 1971).

Studies of chronic ventilator dependence in COPD patients usually focus on the psychological sequelae of extended ventilator support, rather than its psychological antecedents. The neuropsychological functioning of these patients, who are often elderly, varies considerably with the partial pressure of arterial oxygen, and the associated mood changes can seldom be tagged as only causes of or results of the swings in the patient's physical condition. Several psychological complaints are known to be associated with ventilator dependence and include (but are not limited to) fears of death, abandonment, and separation; financial strain; changes in self-image; and mutilation. All can have effects, in the acute setting, on reported respiratory distress, respiratory rate, and perceived work of breathing, and may thereby contribute to the clinical appearance of a new or continued need for mechanical ventilation (LaFond and Horner 1988).

Many investigators have also described the effects of the patient's extended need for mechanical ventilation on the family of the patient. The "ability to cope" is seen as both a patient and a family attribute, and as an indicator of the patient's eventual aptitude for weaning from the ventilator (Sivak et al. 1986). The most successful qualities, or adaptive defense mechanisms, are those that efficiently reduce the conscious experience of anxiety (Ford 1983; J. F. Miller 1983; Strain 1978). Patients and families deal best with the off-again, on-again experience of chronic ventilator existence through attributes of "high motivation," "optimism," "resourcefulness," "flexibility," "pragmatism," and "avoidance of emotional extremes" (Weisman 1987). One wonders what chronically stressful experience would not be better endured by persons with such traits. Educability and a lack of severe preexistent psychopathology are also considered positive long-term prognostic indicators (Gilmartin 1986; Gilmartin and Make 1983).

Rheumatologic Disease

Rheumatoid Arthritis

Rheumatoid arthritis, like asthma, is one of the classic psychosomatic diseases and shares with it many historical characteristics. As in the case of asthma, patients and physicians alike often associate severe psychological stress with the onset of the disease and with its exacerbations.

Some discussion of the pathophysiology may facilitate an understanding of the discussion that follows. The exact etiology of rheumatoid arthritis is unknown, but it is widely held to be an immunologically based disease. Some injury or other event on a microvascular scale is probably the first step in the pathogenetic pathway. Synovial membrane proliferation then occurs as a result of repeated inflammatory responses in the affected tissue. Local antibody production follows, and immune complexes form with the joining of rheumatoid factors and IgGs. Activation of complement follows, with the invasion of intravascular fluid and of cellular components into the joint space. Proteolytic enzymes are released, with destruction of protein and exacerbation of the existent inflammation. Circulating immune complexes may contribute to the pathologic features seen in extra-articular sites (Hardin 1986b).

The strong association of rheumatoid arthritis with human leukocyte antigen DR4 suggests a hereditary predisposition, perhaps one that is a genetic immunologic defect. The association is highest for whites, blacks, Japanese, and Hispanics and is not seen among Jews (M. L. Miller and Glass 1981).

Much of the early psychological work on rheumatoid arthritis was an attempt to define the "rheumatic personality," a profile that conferred on the patient a high risk for contracting the disease or for relapse in patients already afflicted (Halliday 1942). Rheumatoid arthritis patients were seen as self-sacrificing, masochistic, inhibited, perfectionist, and retiring (Moos 1964; Moos and Solomon 1964). Their emotions were "unavailable" to them (Silverman 1985). Female rheumatoid arthritis patients were described as active suppressors of anger and sexuality. Male patients were seen as more depressive. Compared with the general population, one investigator found rheumatoid arthritis patients more "neurotic," more likely to try to be socially pleasing, and at higher risk for psychiatric disturbances (Gardiner 1980). Some investigators, however, found little difference between rheumatoid arthritis patients and a nonpatient population (Cassileth et al. 1984; Crown et al. 1975).

A variety of psychological reactions to rheumatoid arthritis and its sequelae have been described. In many instances, these reactions may go on to contribute to a perpetuation of the relapse or toward a worsening of the patient's condition. Such responses to the disease and to its treatment may include those adaptive and maladaptive styles that affect rehabilitation efforts as well (Kahana and Bibring 1964; Lipowski 1975; Meenan 1981).

Depression may result from an acute awareness of the illness and the losses it imposes on patients, and it impedes the patients' participation in their own care and potential for any recovery of function. On psychological testing 40%–50% of rheumatoid arthritis patients appear depressed (Halliday 1942). Other characteristics of the psychological profiles of rheumatoid arthritis patients resemble those of other groups of chronically ill patients: elevated hypochondriasis, hysteria, and rare elevations of psychotic scales (Polley et al. 1970).

Although there are numerous studies that attest to the central importance of the experience of the loss of mobility (Molodofsky and Chester 1970), especially for the elderly (Rosillo and Vogel 1971), there are no good investigations of therapy for the resulting states of grief. One might wonder, for example, if the treatment of resulting depressive conditions would have a discernible effect on rates of remission or ability to participate in a rehabilitation program.

Other psychological attributes that adversely affect the capacity for rehabilitation in rheumatoid arthritis include poor motivation, "lack of intelligence," dysphoric mood not associated with physical pain, deficient ego strength, and poor impulse control (Molodofsky and Chester 1970; Rosillo and Vogel 1971). A "positive attitude" toward rehabilitation personnel and the view of rehabilitation goals as potentially flexible and adjustable are conducive to a good outcome (Vogel and Rosillo 1971).

The foregoing has been a summary of the phenomenologically based experience with psychological factors affecting the course of rheumatoid arthritis; the studies examine the clinical surface of the disease. At another hierarchical level, rheumatoid arthritis is understood to be a disease mediated through the immune system; autoimmune hyperactivity, the inappropriate direction of the body's defensive efforts against itself, is widely held to be the crucial pathophysiological mechanism. Phenomena suggesting linkage between the immune system and the neurologic system have been widely studied in rheumatoid arthritis patients, in patients with other diseases felt to be immunologically based, and in experimental animals. What follows is a brief survey of some of the conclusions, problems, and questions raised by research in this arena of interdigitating systems—the psychobiological interface. The outcome of this work may eventually have relevance for patients with rheumatoid arthritis and other immunologically based diseases.

The past two decades have seen a surge in research on the effects of positive and negative emotions on human immune functioning. Some disorders reported to result from acute "stress," such as cardiac dysrhythmias and myocardial infarction, are not discernibly involved with immune functioning. Others, which seem to worsen or have their onset after severe stressors, such as infectious mononucleosis, colds, influenza, cancer, and multiple sclerosis, may devolve from complex combinations of immune hyper- and hypofunctioning (Melnechuk 1988).

Over 20 years ago, in their classic study, Holmes and Rahe (1967) described the potential effects of stress on health. The death of a spouse was the life stressor most closely associated with imminent adverse consequences to health; later investigators postulated an immune-mediated mechanism for the finding, at least in part because of the high incidence of cancer as the cause of deterioration of health in the surviving spouses.

Although the trends in research in this area seem to be closing in on a clearer understanding of how the meaning of life events (and their associated emotions) affect immune functioning, one gets the feeling, in reviewing the literature, that we are still a long way from clinical application of recent findings. Studies on "stress" and human cancer, for example, have yielded mixed results; the approaches have lacked experimental consistency and sophistication (Anisman and Zacharko 1983). Early theories about the emotional effects on the body's system of immunosurveillance (and thus, on the incidence of cancer) hinged on the clear elaboration of the immunosurveillance system in a theory of the natural evolution of cancer. The latter connection has now come under attack.

Natural killer cell activity, one arm of the immunosurveillance system and the one probably most significantly connected with tumor control, has been found to have an important (Irwin et al. 1987), although only a weak and nonspecific (Heisel et al. 1986), connection with psychological health. The response to stress, rather than the nature of the stress itself, may be most important in determining the quality and efficacy of the eventual immune response (DeLisi and Crow 1986). Cellular immune functioning has been studied in the context of a number of activities and life events (such as advanced age, sleep deprivation, marathon running, protein-calorie malnutrition, heavy cigarette smoking and alcohol use, and opiate addiction), and the reader is referred elsewhere (Calabrese et al. 1987).

Major claims have been made for the psychoneural modulation of immunity, based on research ranging from the psychological to the molecular in focus (Melnechuk 1988). Several of interest are listed.

1. Immune responses can be suppressed and enhanced by Pavlovian conditioning (Ader 1985).
2. Specific immune functions can be affected by stimulation or destruction of several brain regions (including cerebral cortex, hypothalamus, and midbrain median raphe nuclei). These immune effects are lateralized (Melnechuk 1988; Renoux et al. 1987).
3. Solid tissues of the immune system contain a marker for the diffuse neuroendocrine system and are innervated by the autonomic nervous system. Noradrenergic nerve fibers contact individual lymphocytes in the spleen. The sympathetic nervous system appears to have an inhibiting effect on some types of immune responsiveness: sympathectomy enhances the severity of experimental autoimmune myasthenia gravis (Angeletti and Hickey 1985).
4. Immune solid tissues display receptor molecules for binding many classical polypeptide neurotransmitters and hormones, including those released during distress responses, such as beta-adrenergic agonists, acetylcholine, dopamine, and vasoactive intestinal polypeptide (Angeletti and Hickey 1985).
5. Many neurotransmitters and hormones influence the numbers of and responsiveness of lymphocytes during an immune response (Hall and Goldstein 1985).
6. In a manner similar to that of the neural regulatory system, the hypothalamus and pituitary gland receive feedback messages from the immune system. Ablation of the immune system affects brain waves in the ventromedial hypothalamus and the cerebral cortex (Blalock and Smith 1985; Dafny et al. 1985).
7. More specifically with regard to rheumatoid arthritis, natural experiments in humans suggest autonomic or other neurologic linkage with the immune system: arthritic limbs may improve after denervation. Even in disease of long duration, hemiparetic limbs may be unaffected when the paresis precedes the onset of the rheumatoid arthritis (Rodnan 1973; Silverman 1985).

The relationship between the immune system and the brain is therefore two-way, with many messengers having been proposed as the carriers of information (changes in corticosteroid concentration, prostaglandins, and opiates being examples of specific mediators). Nonspecific mediators might include substances secreted from cells of phagocytic lineage (*Lancet* 1987).

Thus, in the study of psychological factors affecting rheumatoid arthritis, the fight will have to proceed on two fronts: the clinical, where most work has been conducted, but with improvements (some of which are suggested later), and the neuroimmunologic, where some news promises to give us a theoretical underpinning for the anecdotal reports given by physicians and patients for years.

Fibrositis

Fibrositis is a commonly diagnosed, but poorly delineated, entity. Symptoms include widespread myalgia, disturbed sleep, and pain trigger points. There are no reliable diagnostic procedures, although the detection of a trigger point (especially one along the superior border of the trapezius muscle or at the second costochondral junction) may be an approximation. Emotional distress, such as depressed affect, is considered universal among these patients, but one wonders whether this may not at least in part be due to the patients' repeated failures to find satisfactory explanations and treatment for their misery. Anywhere from 10% to 56% of patients have a non–rapid eye movement sleep disorder, manifested as daytime fatigue (Hardin 1986a). Patient selection varies a great deal from study to study, but fibrositis patients seem to demonstrate high levels of depression on psychological testing.

The treatment of the sleep disorder, usually with tricyclic antidepressants, is helpful for most patients (Hardin 1986a). Sedating, serotonergically active agents are often recommended (Goldenberg 1986). Because of this responsiveness, and because of the high prevalence of "depressive characteristics" in first-degree relatives of fibrositis patients (Goldenberg 1986), fibrositis has been called a "depressive equivalent." This somewhat vague term is used in what often seems like an attempt to straddle the confusing territory that fibrositis seems to occupy: the point at which psyche meets soma.

Conclusions and Recommendations

Patients and physicians do not need to be convinced of the interdependent relationship between somatic illness and emotional life, but an understanding of the nature of that linkage could help us be better physicians.

Research in asthma and COPD needs prospective studies that closely examine the temporal sequence of emotional events in the life of the patient and the perturbations of the respective illnesses. COPD research, in particular, should examine more carefully the potential psychological antecedents to exacerbations of COPD, now that so much is known about the psychological sequelae. This is not to say that the door should be closed on the latter, but that the preponderance of effort needs to be directed earlier in the causal chain of events. The search for a reliable and useful animal model in asthma continues and may some day provide the opportunity for closer examination of stress and its effects on the activity of asthma. Increased focus on asthma in twins (among whom severity of illness is often conveniently uniform) prospectively might provide the chance to unlock the issue of the effects of personality structure on the course of the disease.

For rheumatoid arthritis research, the preponderance of retrospective studies, mainly focused on psychological sequelae, is an obvious problem. The recommendations here would be similar to those for asthma researchers. The long-term studies, however, could not begin in childhood because there is no clear-cut childhood equivalent to rheumatoid arthritis. Study protocols that use measurements of rheumatoid factor as an index of disease severity and of responsiveness to psychiatric interventions need a more consistent application of procedure and of nomenclature—for example, more stringent regard for the timing of the sampling of rheumatoid factor with respect to the stressful event, and more careful attention paid to the possible catabolic and anabolic effects on rheumatoid factor by administered drugs, such as corticosteroids.

Immunologically based research (on rheumatoid arthritis and on other diseases) is similarly afflicted; the lack of a consistent nomenclature (e.g., what is to be considered "stress"? *severe* stress?) is a major methodological problem. Social and psychiatric variables end up more poorly defined than immunologic variables. The sampling of stress-related hormones is also unsophisticated with regard to the temporal sequence of events (Melnechuk 1988).

With the design of well-controlled, prospective studies that utilize uniform definitions of stressful psychological events, future researchers may be able to expand our functional understanding of the psychological forces affecting pulmonary and rheumatologic illnesses.

References

Ader R: Behaviorally conditioned modulation of immunity, in Neural Modulation of Immunity. Edited by Guillemin RG, Cohen M, Melnechuk T. New York, Raven, 1985, pp 1–21

Agle DP, Baum GL: Psychological aspects of chronic obstructive pulmonary disease. Med Clin North Am 61:749–758, 1977

Alexander F: Psychosomatic Medicine: Its Principles and Applications. New York, WW Norton, 1950

American Psychiatric Association: Diagnostic and Statistical Manual of Mental Disorders, 4th Edition. Washington, DC, American Psychiatric Association, 1994

Angeletti RH, Hickey WF: A neuroendocrine marker in tissues of the immune system. Science 230:89–90, 1985

Anisman H, Zacharko RM: Stress and neoplasia: speculations and caveats. Behavioral Medicine Update 5:27–35, 1983

Bengtsson U: Emotions and asthma, I. European Journal of Respiratory Disease Suppl 136:123–129, 1984

Blalock JE, Smith EM: A complete regulatory loop between the immune and neuroendocrine systems. Federation Proceedings 44:108–111, 1985

Burns BH, Howell JBL: Disproportionately severe breathlessness in chronic bronchitis. Q J Med 38:277–294, 1969

Calabrese JR, Kling MA, Gold PW: Alterations in immunocompetence during stress, bereavement, and depression: focus on neuroendocrine regulation. Am J Psychiatry 144:1123–1134, 1987

Cassileth BR, Lusk EJ, Strouse TB, et al: Psychological status in chronic illness: a comparative analysis of six diagnostic groups. N Engl J Med 311:506–511, 1984

Clark RJH, Cochrane GM: Effect of personality on alveolar ventilation in patients with chronic airways obstruction. Br Med J 1:273–275, 1970

Crown S, Crown JM, Fleming A: Aspects of the psychology and epidemiology of rheumatoid disease. Psychol Med 5:291–299, 1975

Cugell DW, Fish JE (eds): Beta-2 adrenergic agents and other drugs in reversible airways disease. Chest 73 (suppl):913–1002, 1978

Dafny N, Dougherty P, Pellis NR: The effect of immunosuppression and opiates upon the visual evoked responses of cortical and subcortical structures. Society for Neuroscience Abstracts 11:907, 1985

DeArujo G, Van Arsdel PO, Holmes TH: Life change, coping ability and chronic extrinsic asthma. J Psychosom Res 17:359–363, 1973

DeLisi LE, Crow TJ: Is schizophrenia a viral or immunological disorder? Psychiatr Clin North Am 9:115–132, 1986

Dudley DL, Martin CJ, Holmes TH: Dyspnea: psychological and physiological observations. J Psychosom Res 11:325–339, 1968

Dudley DL, Glaser EM, Jorgenson B, et al: Psychosocial concomitants to rehabilitation in chronic obstructive pulmonary disease, I: psychosocial and psychological considerations. Chest 77:413–420, 1980

Dunbar F: Mind and Body: Psychosomatic Medicine. New York, Random House, 1947

Fishman DB, Petty TL: Physical, symptomatic, and psychological improvement in patients receiving comprehensive care for chronic airway obstruction. J Chronic Dis 24:775–785, 1971

Ford CV: The Somatizing Disorders: Illness as a Way of Life. New York, Elsevier Biomedical, 1983

French TM, Alexander F: Psychogenic factors in bronchial asthma. Psychosomatic Medicine Monographs, Vol 4, 1941, pp 82–101

Friedman MS: Psychological factors associated with pediatric asthma death: a review. J Asthma 21:97–117, 1984

Gantt WAH: Experimental basis for neurotic behavior. Psychosomatic Medicine Monographs, Vol 3, 1944, pp 62–81

Gardiner BM: Psychological aspects of rheumatoid arthritis. Psychol Med 10:159–163, 1980

Geddes DM: Chronic airflow obstruction. Postgrad Med J 60:194–200, 1984

Gilmartin M, Make B: Home care of the ventilator-dependent person. Respiratory Care 28:1490–1497, 1983

Gilmartin ME: Patient and family education. Clin Chest Med 7:619–627, 1986

Goldenberg DL: Psychological studies in fibrositis. Am J Med 81:67–70, 1986

Hall NR, Goldstein AL: Neurotransmitters and host defense, in Neural Modulation of Immunity. Edited by Guillemin RG, Cohen M, Melnechuk T. New York, Raven, 1985, pp 143–156

Halliday JL: Psychological aspects of rheumatoid arthritis. Proceedings of the Royal Society of Medicine 35:455–457, 1942

Hardin JG: Fibrositis, in Clinical Rheumatology. Edited by Ball GV, Koopman WJ. Philadelphia, PA, WB Saunders, 1986a, pp 315–318

Hardin JG: Rheumatoid arthritis, in Clinical Rheumatology. Edited by Ball GV, Koopman WJ. Philadelphia, PA, WB Saunders, 1986b, pp 63–88

Heisel JS, Locke SE, Kraus LJ, et al: Natural killer cell activity and MMPI scores of a cohort of college students. Am J Psychiatry 143:1382–1386, 1986

Holmes TH, Rahe RH: The social adjustment scale. J Psychosom Res 11:213–218, 1967

Hudgel DW, Cooperson DM, Kinsman RA: Recognition of added resistive loads in asthma: the importance of behavioral styles. Am Rev Respir Dis 126:121–125, 1982

Irwin M, Daniels M, Bloom ET, et al: Life events, depressive symptoms, and immune function. Am J Psychiatry 144:437–441, 1987

Kahana RJ, Bibring GL: Personality types in medical management, in Psychiatry and Medical Practice in a General Hospital. Edited by Zinbi RGN. New York, International Universities Press, 1964, pp 108–123

Karol C: The role of primal scene and masochism in asthma. International Journal of Psychoanalytic Psychotherapy 8:577–592, 1980–1981

Knapp PH: The asthmatic and his environment. J Nerv Ment Dis 149:133–151, 1969

Knapp PH, Mathe AA: Psychophysiologic aspects of bronchial asthma: a review, in Bronchial Asthma: Mechanisms and Therapeutics. Edited by Weiss EB, Segal MS, Stein M. Boston, MA, Little, Brown, 1985, pp 914–931

LaFond L, Horner J: Psychosocial issues related to long-term ventilatory support. Problems in Respiratory Care 1:241–256, 1988

Lancet: Depression, stress, and immunity (editorial). Lancet 1:1467–1468, 1987

Lehrer PM, Sargunaraj D, Hochron S: Psychological approaches to the treatment of asthma. J Consult Clin Psychol 60:639–643, 1992

Lipowski ZJ: Physical illness, the patient and his environment: psychosocial foundations of medicine, in American Handbook of Psychiatry, 4th Edition. Edited by Arieti S. Baltimore, MD, Williams & Wilkins, 1975, pp 1263–1277

Mascia A, Frank S, Berkman A, et al: Mortality versus improvement in severe chronic asthma: physiologic and psychologic factors. Ann Allergy 62:311–317, 1989

Mathe AA, Knapp PH: Decreased plasma free fatty acids and urinary epinephrine in bronchial asthma. N Engl J Med 281:234–238, 1969

Meenan RF: The impact of chronic disease: a sociomedical profile of rheumatoid arthritis. Arthritis Rheum 24:544–549, 1981

Melnechuk T: Emotions, brain, immunity, and health: a review, in Emotions and Psychopathology. Edited by Clynes M, Panksepp A. New York, Plenum, 1988, pp 181–248

Miller BD, Strunk RC: Circumstances surrounding the deaths of children due to asthma: a case-control study. Am J Dis Child 143:1294–1299, 1989

Miller JF: Patient power resources, in Coping With Chronic Illness: Overcoming Powerlessness. Edited by Miller JF. Philadelphia, PA, FA Davis, 1983, pp 1–13

Miller ML, Glass DN: The major histocompatibility antigens in rheumatoid arthritis and juvenile arthritis. Bull Rheum Dis 31:21–25, 1981

Molodofsky H, Chester WJ: Pain and mood patterns in patients with rheumatoid arthritis. Psychosom Med 32:309–317, 1970

Moos RH: Personality factors associated with rheumatoid arthritis: a review. J Chronic Dis 17:41–55, 1964

Moos RH, Solomon GF: Personality correlates of the rapidity of progression of rheumatoid arthritis. Ann Rheum Dis 23:145–151, 1964

Plutchik R, Williams MH, Jerrett I, et al: Emotions, personality, and life stresses in asthma. J Psychosom Res 22:425–431, 1978

Polley HF, Swenson WN, Steinhilber R: Personality characteristics of patients with rheumatoid arthritis. Psychosomatics 11:45–49, 1970

Rees L: Physical and emotional factors in bronchial asthma. J Psychosom Res 1:98–114, 1956

Renoux G, Biziere K, Renoux M, et al: Consequences of bilateral brain neocortical ablation on imuthiol-induced immunostimulation in mice. Ann N Y Acad Sci 496:346–353, 1987

Rodnan GP (ed): Primer on rheumatic diseases. JAMA (special issue) 224:662–812, 1973

Rosillo RH, Vogel ML: Correlation of psychological variables and progress in physical rehabilitation, IV: the relation of body image to the success of rehabilitation. Arch Phys Med Rehabil 52:182–186, 1971

Sandhu HS: Psychosocial issues in chronic obstructive pulmonary disease. Clin Chest Med 7:642–649, 1986

Schiavi R, Stein M, Sethi BB: Respiratory variables in response to a pain-fear stimulus and in experimental asthma. Psychosom Med 13:254–261, 1951

Sharma S, Nandkumar VK: Personality structure and adjustment pattern in bronchial asthma. Acta Psychiatr Scand 61:81–88, 1980

Silverman AJ: Rheumatoid arthritis, in Comprehensive Textbook of Psychiatry, 4th Edition. Edited by Kaplan HI, Sadock BJ. Baltimore, MD, Williams & Wilkins, 1985, pp 1185–1198

Sivak ED, Cordasco EM, Gipson GT, et al: Home care ventilation: the Cleveland Clinic experience from 1977 to 1985. Respiratory Care 31:294–301, 1986

Strain JJ: Psychological Intervention in Medical Practice. New York, Appleton-Century-Crofts, 1978

Teiramaa E: Psychic factors and the inception of asthma. J Psychosom Res 23:253–262, 1979

Teiramaa E: Psychosocial factors, personality, and acute-insidious onset asthma. J Psychosom Res 25:43–49, 1981

Tunsater A: Emotions and asthma, II. Eur J Respir Dis Suppl 136:131–137, 1984

Vogel ML, Rosillo RH: Correlation of psychological variables and progress in physical rehabilitation, III: ego functions and defensive and adaptive mechanisms. Arch Phys Med Rehabil 52:15–21, 1971

Weiner H: Psychobiology and Human Disease. New York, Elsevier, 1977

Weiner H: Respiratory disorders, in Comprehensive Textbook of Psychiatry. Edited by Kaplan HE, Freedman AM, Sadock FJ. Baltimore, MD, Williams & Wilkins, 1985, pp 1159–1169

Weisman AD: Coping with illness, in MGH Handbook of General Hospital Psychiatry. Edited by Hackett T, Cassem N. Littleton, MA, PSG Publishing, 1987, pp 297–308

CHAPTER 9

End-Stage Renal Disease

JAMES L. LEVENSON, M.D.
SUSAN GLOCHESKI, M.D.

There has been extensive interest in the psychosocial and psychiatric aspects of dialysis and transplantation paralleling the evolution of treatment approaches to end-stage renal disease (ESRD) (Czaczkes and Kaplan De-Nour 1978; Levy 1981, 1983). In this chapter we review the systematic research literature regarding the influence of psychological factors on the course of chronic renal disease. Topics covered include the prevalence of psychiatric disorders (affective disorders) in ESRD patients and comparison of psychosocial quality of life in ESRD patients receiving different treatment modalities (hemodialysis, peritoneal dialysis, renal transplantation, and home versus center dialysis). Systematic studies of psychological factors affecting outcome in ESRD have focused on depression or noncompliance. Issues of withdrawal from dialysis, mechanisms mediating the effects of psychological factors, and directions for future research are also addressed.

Standard references were reviewed (Czaczkes and Kaplan De-Nour 1978; Levy 1981, 1983, 1987). Only studies that utilized assessment measures of established validity were included. Strict criteria of adequate sample size and adequate control for bias and confounding factors (e.g., disease severity) were not imposed because too small a number of studies would have qualified.

Prevalence of Psychiatric Morbidity

Essentially all of the systematic research on the prevalence of psychopathology in ESRD patients has focused on depression. Early research showed widely varying rates of depression in dialysis patients, from 0% (Wright et al. 1966) to 100% (Reichsman and Levy 1972). One explanation for this discrepancy lies in differences in the definitions and criteria used for depression. For example, in ESRD patients on dialysis, Smith and colleagues (1985) found that the proportion of depressed patients was 47% by the Beck Depression Inventory, 10% by the Multiple Affect Adjective Checklist, and 5% by DSM-III (American Psychiatric Association 1980) criteria. Hinrichsen and colleagues (1989) evaluated in-center hemodialysis patients with the Schedule for Affective Disorders and Schizophrenia and identified 17.7% meeting criteria for minor depression and 6.5% meeting criteria for major depression as defined by Research Diagnostic Criteria (Spitzer et al. 1978).

In a group of hemodialysis and peritoneal dialysis patients, all of whom had been treated for at least 3 months, Craven and colleagues (1987) found that 8.1% met DSM-III criteria for major depression and that 6.1% met criteria for dysthymic disorder. Lowry and Atcherson (1980) evaluated patients who were just beginning home-based dialysis and found that 18% met DSM-III criteria for depression. All of these prevalence rates are higher than those found in community-based samples—such as the Epidemiologic Catchment Area study (Regier et al. 1984)—but most do not appear higher than rates generally found in patients with other chronic medical illnesses (Katon and Sullivan 1990).

There are a number of serious difficulties in comparing these studies with each other or in generalizing from them. Some focused on a single modality and site of treatment (e.g., in-center hemodialysis), whereas others used mixed groups. This makes interpretation difficult because differences in psychosocial adjustment have been demonstrated between patients receiving different modalities of treatment for ESRD (see below). Some studies measured the point prevalence of psychiatric disorders, whereas others assessed lifetime history. Some investigators assessed patients early in the course of dialysis, others much later, and some made no attempt to standardize when the patient was studied in relation to the onset of dialysis. Such lack of standardization can create prevalence-incidence (Neyman) bias (Levenson et al. 1990). It is also well recognized by nephrologists and psychiatrists that psychological adjustment substantially varies over the course of ESRD treatment (Kutner et al.

1985). Differences in demographics (e.g., race, sex, age) as well as in location (e.g., academic medical center versus community based, urban versus rural) should be noted, but such factors are not always well described.

There are additional problems that have not been adequately addressed in studies of the prevalence of depression in ESRD. Somatic symptoms are strongly associated with depressed affect in dialysis patients (Barrett et al. 1990), but the direction of causality remains unclear. Uremia itself produces irritability, decreased appetite, insomnia, depressed sensorium, apathy, fatigue, and poor concentration. Dialyzed patients vary in the degree to which uremia is successfully corrected. Therefore, some depressive symptoms in the ESRD population may represent incompletely treated uremia rather than depression (Hart and Kreutzer 1988). Furthermore, ESRD patients as a group have many other conditions that may mimic depressive states or cause organic mood disorders, including anemia, electrolyte disturbances, and underlying systemic disease (e.g., systemic lupus erythematosus). Patients may also take medications with depressive side effects, including antihypertensives, corticosteroids, anti-inflammatory agents, metoclopramide, and sedative-hypnotics. Some studies have addressed these potential confounding factors by modifying structured diagnostic instruments to discount somatic symptoms attributable to medical illness or to drugs, for example (Hinrichsen et al. 1989).

Quality of Life: Which Treatment Is Best?

A number of studies have compared psychosocial quality of life with dialysis versus renal transplantation. Evans and colleagues (1985) found that 79% of transplant recipients functioned psychosocially at nearly normal levels, compared with 47%–59% of dialysis patients. Transplant recipients had better quality of life than dialysis patients on both objective and subjective measures. All of the differences in quality of life persisted after the patient case mix was controlled for differences in demographics and medical characteristics. Petrie (1989) found that dialysis patients showed more morbidity on the General Health Questionnaire (mainly loss of emotional control and depression) compared with transplant patients and healthy control subjects. Australian (Morris and Jones 1989) and German (Zimmermann 1989) reports also confirmed better quality of life in renal transplantation. Similar results have been demonstrated in pediatric ESRD (Brownbridge and Fielding 1991; Reynolds et al. 1991). On the other hand, Kalman and colleagues (1983) found no difference in psychiatric morbidity between dialysis and transplant patients, even though in their study the former were older and medically more ill. In a comparison of 31 transplant recipients and 31 dialysis patients matched for duration of treatment, age, education, and family status, psychological adjustment was similar in the two groups (Sayag et al. 1990). Finally, we should note that such studies usually do not address the effects of transplant failure, which may result in the worst quality of life (Bremer et al. 1989).

Investigators also have compared the quality of life between patients receiving different dialysis modalities. Wolcott and colleagues (1988) found that continuous ambulatory peritoneal dialysis (CAPD) patients had better quality of life and better cognitive functioning than hemodialysis patients, with the differences explained neither medically nor demographically, and there have been similar findings in children with renal failure (Brownbridge and Fielding 1991). Others have found little or no difference in psychosocial outcomes between hemodialysis and CAPD patients (Evans et al. 1985; Soskolne and Kaplan De-Nour 1987). Comparison of hemodialysis or CAPD at a hospital versus dialysis at home has shown treatment at home to appear psychosocially superior, but the magnitude of difference has varied (Evans et al. 1985; Soskolne and Kaplan De-Nour 1987).

These quality-of-life studies have methodological limitations that hinder comparison and interpretation. A fundamental problem is that ESRD patients are never randomized to receive a particular form of dialysis or transplantation; indeed, bias in treatment assignment is well recognized (Kjellstrand et al. 1989; Smith et al. 1983). Thus, any outcome differences may be related to pretreatment differences in medical, psychosocial, rehabilitative, or demographic characteristics. The most recent studies have attempted to correct for this statistically, but it cannot be entirely corrected. This point is exemplified in a study of 459 ESRD patients that included four modalities of treatment: in-center hemodialysis, CAPD, related transplant, and cadaver transplant (Julius et al. 1989). Differences in quality of life were demonstrated, but when the investigators adjusted for demographics, primary cause of ESRD, and comorbid illness, they found a reduction in the significance of differences among the four treatment modalities, as well as a change in the quality-of-life rank order.

Psychological Factors and Outcome Studies

There are a number of potential measures that can be studied in ESRD, including survival, adequacy of dialysis and dietary compliance (as assessed by blood urea nitrogen, creatinine, potassium, phosphate, interdialytic weight gain, blood pressure, and other tests), and complications (bone disease, access problems, infection, pericarditis, and other disorders). Functional outcome measures include various indices of quality of life, health care utilization, employment, and family stability.

Depression

A Canadian research group (Burton et al. 1986; Richmond et al. 1982; Wai et al. 1981) studied the relationship between psychosocial factors and survival in 285 home hemodialysis patients. They found that depression (on the Basic Personality Inventory) was a better predictor of (shorter) survival than was age or a composite physiological index that included 19 chemical and clinical variables (Burton et al. 1986). Numan and colleagues (1981) found that depressive symptoms (on the Depression Adjective Check List) were associated with higher mortality and more frequent hospitalization in 53 hemodialysis patients, who had been on dialysis from 0 to 150 months. Ziarnik and colleagues (1977) studied 47 in-center hemodialysis patients and found that those who died within the first year were more likely to have been depressed (on a Minnesota Multiphasic Personality Inventory administered prior to beginning hemodialysis) than those who survived longer. Shulman and colleagues (1989) examined mortality at 10-year follow-up in 64 center and home dialysis patients and found that age and depressive symptoms (on the Beck Depression Inventory) were better predictors of survival than medical variables.

A fundamental weakness of most of these studies is that no attempt is made to measure or to control for disease severity, so the findings simply could be the result of patients who are more ill being more likely to get depressed. Disease severity is a common confounding factor in studies of psychopathology in the medically ill (Levenson et al. 1990). A number of general measures of disease severity are available (Aronow 1988), and a measure developed specifically for ESRD, which has good reliability and validity, has been reported (Craven et al. 1991)

Other studies have not supported the relationship between depression and decreased survival time in ESRD. Devins and colleagues (1990) studied a mixed group of 97 patients (hemodialysis, CAPD, transplant) and found no effects of depression on survival. Indeed, in their study those patients who described their lives as happy overall had the shortest survival times, leaving the authors to speculate about denial. In a study of 78 hemodialysis and CAPD patients over age 70 years, Husebye and colleagues (1987) also found no relationship between depressive symptoms (Likert Scale) and survival.

No published studies were found examining relationships between psychological factors and outcome in renal transplantation, with the exception of studies that were too small to provide meaningful findings (Keegan et al. 1983). Fortunately, large, long-term studies are underway (Wilson 1990). Psychosocial intervention outcome studies in ESRD mostly have been nonrandomized and uncontrolled or poorly controlled. In a naturalistic, nonrandomized design, Friend and colleagues (1986) investigated the effects of participation in a support group by dialysis patients compared with control subjects. They found that support-group participants lived longer than nonparticipants, even after controlling for 13 psychosocial and physiological covariates. This study must be interpreted cautiously in view of the nonrandomized design as well as the lack of records indicating when patients joined the group and how long they attended.

Compliance

Psychosocial factors with demonstrated effects on compliance in ESRD include patients' beliefs about their health behaviors (Cummings et al.

1982), "locus of control" and self-efficacy (Schneider et al. 1991), family problems (Cummings et al. 1982), and social support (O'Brien 1990). Studies of compliance in dialysis patients have many of the same methodological problems as those focusing on depression. Particularly problematic has been the question of how to define and measure noncompliance. Some studies have used patients' reports or physicians' and nurses' impressions; others have used chart review of interdialytic weight gain and blood chemistry changes. Manley and Sweeney (1986) argued that the cutoffs that have been set impressionistically and used to define compliance have tended to inflate the amount of estimated noncompliance.

Cummings and colleagues (1982) examined which psychosocial factors have the greatest effect on compliance. They found that patients' beliefs about the efficacy of, and barriers to, compliance behavior, as well as reported family problems, were consistent predictors of the degree of compliance. However, this finding held more consistently for subjective rather than objective compliance. In a well-designed study of the effects of family process variables on the survival of center hemodialysis patients, Reiss and colleagues (1986) examined 23 families in a family study laboratory setting. In contrast to expectations, high scores on family problem solving, as well as on measures of accomplishment and intactness (including intelligence, income, and occupational status), predicted early death rather than survival. Patient noncompliance accounted for most of the association between the family variables and survival. Although the relationship found in this study between noncompliance and survival is consistent with other work, the association of noncompliance and early death with indicators of *higher* family functioning is so contrary to clinical experience that the findings should be interpreted with skepticism, particularly considering the small sample size. Overall, although the effects of noncompliance on dialysis patients' outcomes are well recognized by clinicians, they remain insufficiently empirically characterized.

Small studies in kidney transplant patients have shown that pretransplant noncompliance predicts posttransplant noncompliance and graft failure (Rodriguez et al. 1991). Noncompliant kidney transplant patients are more likely to be depressed and have other psychosocial problems than are compliant patients (Rodriguez et al. 1991).

Withdrawal From Dialysis

Psychiatric consultation may be requested when long-term dialysis patients wish to discontinue treatment. Our comments are limited to empirical studies; readers are referred elsewhere for discussion of clinical (Greene 1983), liaison (Slevin 1983), and ethical (Holley et al. 1989) issues. Neu and Kjellstrand (1986) quantified withdrawal from dialysis in a sample of 1,766 ESRD patients who entered a dialysis program between 1966 and 1983. Dialysis was discontinued in 9%, accounting for 22% of all deaths. Half of the patients withdrawn were incompetent, requiring surrogate decision making. The authors asserted that only 3 of the 155 withdrawals from dialysis represented suicide, but this may be an underestimate because no psychiatric evaluation was reported. Similar smaller studies have appeared from Canada (Hirsch 1989) and the Netherlands (van Nieuwkerk et al. 1990). Early studies that had pointed to a very high rate of suicide in dialysis patients overestimated suicide prevalence by not distinguishing rational treatment withdrawal from suicide. The true rate of suicide in dialysis has not been established systematically; nor has there been careful attention to the psychological factors that may affect the decision to withdraw from treatment.

Mechanisms Mediating the Effects
of Psychological Factors

The current state of research allows only for speculation on *how* psychological factors might assert influence over outcome in ESRD. We restrict our comments to the potential influences of depression. Depression has been shown to affect immune function, although the clinical significance of these effects is not yet clear (Stein et al. 1991). It is at least possible that depression-induced immunologic changes might lead to increased infections in dialysis and transplant patients. A much less theoretical explanation, and one familiar to clinicians, is that depressed ESRD patients seem more likely to evidence poor self-care, noncompliance (dietary, medication, dialysis), and poor medical follow-up. Depression may be associated with poor social support in ESRD patients (Siegal et al. 1987), which has its own adverse impact on medical outcome, although this relationship has not been clearly established in ESRD (Burton et al. 1983). Depression has been associated in other populations with increased use of analgesics, which in turn have been demonstrated to have a role in the etiology and exacerbation of chronic renal failure (Sandler et al. 1989; Schwarz et al. 1989). Depression is associated with smoking, alcoholism, and other forms of substance abuse that are themselves major causes of increased morbidity and mortality. Depression may adversely impact outcome in ESRD by serving as a risk factor for other medical comorbidity (e.g., myocardial infarction [Booth-Kewley and Friedman 1987] or reduced aerobic capacity [Carney et al. 1986]). Finally, it is possible that adverse effects of depression in patients with chronic renal failure are nonspecific because depression may be independently associated with increased mortality in the population at large (Murphy et al. 1987).

Future Research

Psychonephrology is an important frontier for research exploring the effects of psychological factors on physical conditions, and much groundbreaking work has been accomplished. Further research with careful attention to methodology is needed to demonstrate and quantify more clearly the effects of psychological factors on renal disease. Although it would be impossible to control all potential confounding factors (Table 9–1), future researchers should make greater attempts to control for differences in demographics, treatment modality, time point in treatment, primary cause of renal failure, other medical and psychiatric comorbidities, smoking, substance abuse, medications, and other relevant factors. Comparisons over time must take into account changes in treatment that also affect emotional status and quality of life (e.g., erythropoietin [Canadian Erythropoietin Study Group 1990]).

Surprisingly, there do not appear to have been any psychiatric studies of chronic renal failure prior to the end stage when dialysis or transplantation are required, although there are large numbers of such patients medically followed for years. Such patients, in fact, have been the subject of a number of studies examining the progression of renal failure as a function of dietary protein intake (Ihle et al. 1989) and blood pressure

TABLE 9–1.　Potential confounding factors in end-stage renal disease

Factors that may affect course of illness	Common adverse events
Blood pressure control	Access infection
Degree of uremia	Access malfunction
Interdialytic weight gain	Graft rejection
Compliance	**Treatment modality**
Calcium/phosphorus metabolism	Hemodialysis
Coexisting systemic disease (e.g., diabetes mellitus, peripheral vascular disease, coronary artery disease)	Hemofiltration
	Peritoneal dialysis
Etiology of renal disease	Transplantation
Duration of illness at the time of study	**Site of treatment**
Anemia	In center
Pruritis	Home
Chronic pain	
Medication side effects (e.g., antihypertensives)	

control (Brazy et al. 1989). Depression and noncompliance would be very interesting cofactors to examine in pre-ESRD patients. The interaction between depression and noncompliance in all forms of treatment for ESRD remains an important area for future research. Controlled intervention trials for treatment of depression, examining medical, psychiatric, and health services outcomes, would be valuable. Finally, studies using structured psychiatric assessment of patients who withdraw from treatment are overdue; such research could better delineate the relative roles of psychopathology and rational decision making.

References

American Psychiatric Association: Diagnostic and Statistical Manual of Mental Disorders, 3rd Edition. Washington, DC, American Psychiatric Association, 1980

Aronow DB: Severity-of-illness measurement: applications in quality assurance and utilization review. Medical Care Review 45:339–366, 1988

Barrett BJ, Vavasour HM, Major A: Clinical and psychological correlates of somatic symptoms in patients on dialysis. Nephron 55:10–15,1990

Booth-Kewley S, Friedman HS: Psychological predictors of heart disease: a quantitative review. Psychol Bull 101:343–362, 1987

Brazy PC, Stead WW, Fitzwilliam JF: Progression of renal insufficiency: role of blood pressure. Kidney Int 35:670–674, 1989

Bremer BA, McCauley CR, Wrona RM, et al: Quality of life in end-stage renal disease: a reexamination. Am J Kidney Dis 13:200–209, 1989

Brownbridge G, Fielding DM: Psychosocial adjustment to end-stage renal failure: comparing hemodialysis, continuous ambulatory peritoneal dialysis and transplantation. Pediatric Nephrology 5:612–616, 1991

Burton HJ, Lindsay RM, Kline SA: Social support as a mediator of psychological dysfunctioning and a determinant of renal failure outcomes. Clinical and Experimental Dialysis and Apheresis 7:371–389, 1983

Burton HJ, Kline SA, Lindsay RM, et al: The relationship of depression to survival in chronic renal failure. Psychosom Med 48:261–269, 1986

Canadian Erythropoietin Study Group: Association between recombinant human erythropoietin and quality of life and exercise capacity of patients receiving haemodialysis. BMJ 300:573–578, 1990

Carney RM, Wetzel RD, Hagberg J, et al: The relationship between depression and aerobic capacity in hemodialysis patients. Psychosom Med 48:143–147, 1986

Craven JL, Rodin GM, Johnson L, et al: The diagnosis of major depression in renal dialysis patients. Psychosom Med 49:482–492, 1987

Craven J, Littlefield C, Rodin G, et al: The Endstage Renal Disease Severity Index (ESRD-SI). Psychol Med 21:237–243, 1991

Cummings K, Becker M, Kirscht J, et al: Psychosocial factors affecting adherence to medical regimens in a group of hemodialysis patients. Med Care 20:567–580, 1982

Czaczkes JW, Kaplan De-Nour A: Chronic Hemodialysis as a Way of Life. New York, Brunner/Mazel, 1978

Devins GM, Mann J, Mandin H, et al: Psychosocial predictor of survival in end-stage renal disease. J Nerv Ment Dis 178:127–133, 1990

Evans RW, Manninen DL, Garrison LP, et al: The quality of life of patients with end-stage renal disease. N Engl J Med 312:553–559, 1985

Friend R, Singletary Y, Mendell N, et al: Group participation and survival among patients with end-stage renal disease. Am J Public Health 76:670–672, 1986

Greene WA: Problems in discontinuation of hemodialysis, in Psychonephrology 2: Psychological Problems in Kidney Failure and Their Treatment. Edited by Levy NB. New York, Plenum, 1983, pp 131–144

Hart RP, Kreutzer JS: Renal system, in Medical Neuropsychology: The Impact of Disease on Behavior. Edited by Tarter RE, Van Thiel DH, Edwards KL. New York, Plenum, 1988, pp 99–120

Hinrichsen GA, Lieberman JA, Pollack S, et al: Depression in hemodialysis patients. Psychosomatics 30:284–289, 1989

Hirsch DJ: Death from dialysis termination. Nephrol Dial Transplant 4:41–44, 1989

Holley JL, Finucane TE, Moss AH: Dialysis patients' attitudes about cardiopulmonary resuscitation and stopping dialysis. Am J Nephrol 9:245–251, 1989

Husebye DG, Westlie L, Styrovoky TJ, et al: Psychological, social, and somatic prognostic indicators in old patients undergoing long-term dialysis. Arch Intern Med 147:1921–1924, 1987

Ihle BU, Becker GJ, Whitworth JA, et al: The effect of protein restriction on the progression of renal insufficiency. N Engl J Med 321:1771–1777, 1989

Julius M, Hawthorne VM, Carpenter-Alting P, et al: Independence in activities of daily living for end-stage renal disease patients: biomedical and demographic correlates. Am J Kidney Dis 13:61–69, 1989

Kalman TP, Wilson PG, Kalman CM: Psychiatric morbidity in long-term renal transplant recipients and patients undergoing hemodialysis. JAMA 250:55–58, 1983

Katon W, Sullivan MD: Depression and chronic medical illness. J Clin Psychiatry 51 (suppl 6):3–11, 1990

Keegan DL, Shipley C, Dineen D, et al: Adjustment to renal transplantation. Psychosomatics 24:825–828, 831, 1983

Kjellstrand CM, Ericsson F, Traneus A, et al: The wish for renal transplantation. ASAIO Trans 35:619–621, 1989

Kutner NG, Fair PL, Kutner MH: Assessing depression and anxiety in chronic dialysis patients. J Psychosom Res 29:23–31, 1985

Levenson JL, Colenda C, Larson DB, et al: Methodology in consultation-liaison research: a classification of biases. Psychosomatics 31:367–376, 1990

Levy NB (ed): Psychonephrology, 1: Psychological Factors in Hemodialysis and Transplantation. New York, Plenum, 1981

Levy NB (ed): Psychonephrology, 2: Psychological Problems in Kidney Failure and Their Treatment. New York, Plenum, 1983

Levy NB: Chronic renal disease, dialysis, and transplantation, in Principles of Medical Psychiatry. Edited by Stoudemire A, Fogel BS. Orlando, FL, Grune & Stratton, 1987, pp 583–594

Lowry MR, Atcherson E: A short-term follow-up of patients with depressive disorder on entry into home dialysis training. J Affective Disord 2:219–227, 1980

Manley M, Sweeney J: Assessment of compliance in hemodialysis adaptation. J Psychosom Res 30:153–161, 1986

Morris PL, Jones B: Life satisfaction across treatment methods for patients with end-stage renal failure. Med J Aust 150:428–432, 1989

Murphy JM, Monson RR, Olivier DC, et al: Affective disorders and mortality: a general population study. Arch Gen Psychiatry 44:473–480, 1987

Neu S, Kjellstrand CM: Stopping long-term dialysis: an empirical study of withdrawal of life-supporting treatment. N Engl J Med 314:14–20, 1986

Numan IM, Barklind KS, Lubin B: Correlates of depression in chronic dialysis patients: morbidity and mortality. Res Nurs Health 4:295–297, 1981

O'Brien ME: Compliance behavior and long-term maintenance dialysis. Am J Kidney Dis 15:209–214, 1990

Petrie K: Psychological well-being and psychiatric disturbance in dialysis and renal transplant patients. Br J Med Psychol 62:91–96, 1989

Regier DA, Myers JK, Kramer M, et al: The NIMH Epidemiologic Catchment Area program: historical context, major objectives, and study populations characteristics. Arch Gen Psychiatry 41:934–941, 1984

Reichsman F, Levy NB: Problems in adaptation to maintenance hemodialysis: a four-year study of 25 patients. Arch Intern Med 130:859–865, 1972

Reiss D, Gonzalez S, Kramer N: Family process, chronic illness, and death. Arch Gen Psychiatry 43:795–804, 1986

Reynolds JM, Garralda ME, Postlethwaite RJ, et al: Changes in psychosocial adjustment after renal transplantation. Arch Dis Child 66:509–513, 1991

Richmond JM, Lindsay RM, Burton HJ, et al: Psychological and physiological factors predicting the outcome on home hemodialysis. Clin Nephrol 17:109–113, 1982

Rodriguez A, Diaz M, Colon A, et al: Psychosocial profile of noncompliant transplant patients. Transplant Proc 23:1807–1809, 1991

Sandler DP, Smith JC, Weinberg CR, et al: Analgesic use and chronic renal disease. N Engl J Med 320:1238–1243, 1989

Sayag R, Kaplan De-Nour A, Shapire Z, et al: Comparison of psychosocial adjustment of male nondiabetic kidney transplant and hospital hemodialysis patients. Nephron 54:214–218, 1990

Schneider MS, Friend R, Whitaker P, et al: Fluid noncompliance and symptomatology in end-stage renal disease: cognitive and emotional variables. Health Psychol 10:209–215, 1991

Schwarz A, Kunzendorf U, Keller F, et al: Progression of renal failure in analgesic-associated nephropathy. Nephron 53:244–249, 1989

Shulman R, Price JD, Spinelli J: Biopsychosocial aspects of long-term survival on end-stage renal failure therapy. Psychol Med 19:945–954, 1989

Siegal BR, Calsyn RJ, Cuddihee RM: The relationship of social support to psychological adjustment in end-stage renal disease patients. Journal of Chronic Disease 40:337–344, 1987

Slevin SE: Termination of hemodialysis treatment: staff reactions, in Psychonephrology 2: Psychological Problems in Kidney Failure and Their Treatment. Edited by Levy NB. New York, Plenum, 1983, pp 117–130

Smith MD, Hong BA, Michelman JE, et al: Treatment bias in the management of end-stage renal disease. Am J Kidney Dis 3:21–26, 1983

Smith MD, Hong BA, Robson AM: Diagnosis of depression in patients with end-stage renal disease. Am J Med 79:160–166, 1985

Soskolne V, Kaplan De-Nour A: Psychosocial adjustment of home hemodialysis, continuous ambulatory peritoneal dialysis and hospital dialysis patients and their spouses. Nephron 47:266–273, 1987

Spitzer RL, Endicott J, Robins E: Research Diagnostic Criteria: rationale and reliability. Arch Gen Psychiatry 35:773–782, 1978

Stein M, Miller AH, Trestman RL: Depression, the immune system, and health and illness: findings in search of meaning. Arch Gen Psychiatry 48:171–177, 1991

van Nieuwkerk CM, Krediet RT, Arisz L: Vrijwillige beeindiging van dialysebe handeling door chronische dialysepatienten [Voluntary discontinuation of dialysis treatment by chronic dialysis patients]. Ned Tijdschr Geneeskd 134:1549–1552, 1990

Wai L, Richmond J, Burton HJ, et al: Influence of psychosocial factors on survival of home-dialysis patients. Lancet 2:1155–1156, 1981

Wilson P: Psychological risk factors in kidney transplantation. Paper presented at the First Working Conference on the Psychiatric, Psychosocial and Ethical Aspects of Organ Transplantation, Toronto, June 9, 1990

Wolcott DL, Wellisch DK, Marsh JT, et al: Relationship of dialysis modality and other factors to cognitive function in chronic dialysis patients. Am J Kidney Dis 12:275–284, 1988

Wright RG, Sand P, Livingston G: Psychological stress during hemodialysis for chronic renal failure. Ann Intern Med 64:611–621, 1966

Ziarnik J, Freeman CW, Sherrard DJ, et al: Psychological correlates of survival on renal dialysis. J Nerv Ment Dis 164:210–213, 1977

Zimmermann E: Lebensqualitat wahrend Nierenersatztherapie [Quality of life in artificial kidney therapy]. Wien Klin Wochenschr 101:780–784, 1989

CHAPTER 10

Endocrine Diseases

GALE BEARDSLEY, M.D.
MICHAEL G. GOLDSTEIN, M.D.

In this chapter the research that has explored the relationship between psychological factors and the onset, exacerbation, and perpetuation of endocrine diseases is reviewed. Such research has focused primarily on three diseases: diabetes mellitus, Graves' disease, and Cushing's disease. The effects of psychological factors on other endocrine disorders have received only scant attention. Research within the emerging area of neuroendocrinology is not specifically reviewed here, although studies that focus on the physiology of the neuroendocrine response will undoubtedly shed light on the relationships between psychological factors and neuroendocrine function. Also, we do not review the extensive literature on the relationship between endocrine disorders and the development and exacerbation of psychiatric disorders and neuropsychiatric symptoms.

Diabetes Mellitus

Psychological Factors Affecting Onset of Illness

Several investigators have looked at the relationship between psychological factors and the onset of diabetes mellitus. Thomas Willis (1684) wrote the following about diabetes mellitus in the 17th century: "Sadness, or long sorrow, as like convulsions, and other depressions and disorders of the animal spirits are used to generate or foment this morbid

173

disposition." Maudsley (1899), Menninger (1935), and Dunbar (1943) speculated that diabetes mellitus is caused by mental anxiety. However, early studies that attempted to show that acute or chronic stress is a cause of diabetes mellitus are significantly flawed because of small numbers of subjects, inadequate control groups, or poor experimental design. Because of these flaws, their conclusion that there is a causal relationship between stress and the onset of diabetes mellitus is suspect.

More recently, a retrospective study gave support to the idea that stressful life events could become triggering factors in the etiology of insulin-dependent diabetes mellitus (IDDM). Robinson and Fuller (1985) examined 13 newly diagnosed diabetic patients, ages 17–34, as well as the siblings of diabetic patients and neighborhood control subjects. By use of a reliable interview instrument, information was gathered about the 3-year period preceding the diagnosis of IDDM. The diabetic patients had a higher frequency (77%) of one or more severe life events prior to diagnosis compared with their disease-free siblings (39%) and age- and gender-matched control subjects (15%). There was also a higher percentage of diabetic patients (54%) who had two or more severe life events prior to diagnosis compared with siblings (8%) and neighborhood control subjects (8%). A Swedish study of 338 children with IDDM and 500 matched control subjects found no difference between these groups in the total frequency of life events in the year prior to diagnosis (Hagglof et al. 1991). However, in children 5–9 years old, events related specifically to actual or threatened losses within the family were significantly more frequent in the diabetic children compared with control subjects (relative risk = 1.82). The relative risk was significantly increased even when controlled for age, gender, and social status. This study suggests that qualitative characteristics of "stress," such as the meaning of a life event or when it occurs, may be more important than the frequency of life events in understanding the relationship between stress and the onset of diabetes.

In contrast, other studies have found no evidence of a causal relationship between stressful life events and diabetes mellitus. Gendel and Benjamin (1946) studied hospitalized military patients and found insufficient evidence to show that stress had caused diabetes mellitus. In retrospective studies such as these, it is difficult to determine whether a stressful event preceded the illness or vice versa. However, a large prospective study

(Cobb and Rose 1973) of air traffic controllers demonstrated no increased risk of developing diabetes mellitus during a 2-year period. In this study, the air traffic controllers were matched to a group of men who were functioning in jobs that did not require rapid decision making and high levels of responsibility.

Our review of the available literature indicates that there is insufficient evidence to support the position that psychological factors directly affect the onset of diabetes mellitus. Additional prospective studies of patients at risk for diabetes with larger numbers of subjects and with improved methodology are necessary before a more definitive statement can be made. In a review article, Helz and Templeton (1990) concluded that researchers have not been able to determine whether psychological factors have a causal role or whether they are effects of the illness. In the following section we discuss the relationship between psychological factors and the course of diabetes mellitus.

Psychological Factors Affecting Course of Illness

Relationship between stress and the course of diabetes. There have been several studies investigating the relationship between psychological factors and metabolic control of glucose in patients with diabetes mellitus. Investigators have hypothesized that psychological factors may affect metabolic control directly by affecting neuroendocrine target organs. However, psychological factors can also affect compliance with recommendations about diet, activity, self-monitoring of glucose control, and medication (Balfour et al. 1993; Helz and Templeton 1990). The results of studies that have not controlled for compliance must be interpreted with caution.

In addition, several early studies have other methodological problems. Early measures of glucose control, such as glucose and ketone levels in urine and blood, episodes of ketoacidosis, insulin requirements, frequency of clinic visits, and serum triglycerides and cholesterol, were relatively unreliable. More recently, glycosylated hemoglobin, a more reliable measure of metabolic control, has been used. Other studies (Hinkle and Wolf 1952; Hinkle et al. 1959; MacGillivray et al. 1981; Schless and von Laveran-Stiebar 1964; Vandenbergh et al. 1966, 1967) have been criticized for such methodological deficiencies as the pooling of IDDM and non-IDDM patients in the same study, the use of a population of highly selected patients, poor definition of experimental conditions, and failure to standardize the stressful situation used as the experimental manipulation.

A study by Kemmer and colleagues (1986) attempted to avoid these previous shortcomings in their examination of the effects of acute stress on metabolic control of glucose in 18 subjects. Three groups—healthy control subjects, normoglycemic patients with IDDM, and hyperglycemic patients with IDDM—were matched according to age, weight, gender, and socioeconomic status. Each subject was exposed to two stressors: 45 minutes of mental arithmetic and 5 minutes of public speaking. All subjects experienced similar increases in heart rate, blood pressure, plasma epinephrine levels, and plasma norepinephrine levels. Plasma cortisol rose significantly after public speaking in all groups. Neither stressor caused significant changes in circulating levels of glucose, ketones, free fatty acids, glucagon, or growth hormone in patients or control subjects. The authors concluded that sudden, short-lived psychological stresses are not likely to affect metabolic control in IDDM even though they produce changes in cardiovascular responses and moderate elevations in plasma catecholamines and cortisol. In a review of studies that have examined the relationship between acute laboratory-induced stress and blood glucose, Goetsch (1989) provided further insight into methodological problems associated with this type of research.

Two studies have shown support for the hypothesis that psychological stress is associated with changes in glucose control in at least a subset of IDDM patients. The research of Halford and colleagues (1990) and Gonder-Frederick and colleagues (1990) both used within-subject design and analytic strategies. Both groups found that some individuals are more metabolically sensitive to stressors than others.

The work of Halford and colleagues (1990) involved 15 IDDM patients who self-monitored psychological stress, diet, exercise, insulin dose, and blood glucose levels over 8 weeks. At the beginning of the study, the subjects completed the Hassles Scale and the Recent Life Changes Questionnaire; glycosylated hemoglobin concentrations were also calculated. There were no statistically significant correlations between glycosylated hemoglobin levels, daily hassles scores, and life events scores. However, 7 of 15 subjects had statistically significant associations between measures of daily psychological stress and blood glucose levels.

Using a closed-loop insulin/glucose infusion system, Gonder-Frederick and colleagues (1990) monitored continuous blood glucose as they exposed 14 subjects with IDDM to two 20-minute standardized stressors and a control condition during two laboratory sessions 12 weeks apart. The "active" stressor involved doing mental arithmetic, the "passive" stressor was watching a disturbing drivers education film, and the control condition was listening to a comedy record album of the subject's choice. Gonder-Frederick and colleagues found significant changes of greater than 17 mg/dl in the glucose levels of 8 of 14 subjects when they were exposed to the active stressor during the first laboratory session. Significant changes in blood glucose levels were not found during the second laboratory sessions, apparently reflecting the development of habituation. The passive stress and control conditions did not produce statistically significant change in blood glucose levels during either session.

These findings contrast with those of Kemmer and colleagues (1986) and most likely reflect differences in the study design. Although Halford and colleagues (1990) and Gonder-Frederick and colleagues (1990) reported data for individual subjects, Kemmer and colleagues compared blood glucose values across subjects, time intervals, and stressor conditions. The within-subject approach of Halford and colleagues and Gonder-Frederick and colleagues, despite relatively small sample sizes, suggests that some individuals are more vulnerable to the effects of stress than others. If this is true, it would be useful to learn more about how respondents differ from nonrespondents.

Because stress is the psychological factor most often studied, it is important to note that there is a trade-off between studying the effects of reliable laboratory stressors that are not very applicable to daily life (e.g., mental arithmetic and public speaking) and those stressors that may be more applicable but less reliable (e.g., stress interviews, daily hassles). Also, the study of the effects of acute stress in a laboratory paradigm leaves the question of the effects of chronic stress unanswered. In a study of 65 young female diabetic patients (Balfour et al. 1993), an interaction between "perceived stress" and dietary disinhibition on metabolic control was uncovered. Glucose control was poorest in women who perceived their lives as stressful and who also reported moderate to high dietary disinhibition. However, blood glucose control was unrelated to stress in women who reported low levels of disinhibition.

Lloyd and colleagues (1991) published the results of a prospective study of 130 adult IDDM and non-IDDM patients. The presence of severe life events and difficulties was not significantly associated with premature death or the development of macrovascular disease over the 4 years of follow-up. However, those who began antihypertensive therapy during the follow-up period were significantly more likely to have experienced five or more severe life events during the previous 5 years than those who did not begin antihypertensive therapy. This relationship was not mediated by baseline blood pressure, type of diabetes, gender, or ethnicity. Clearly, more prospective studies are needed to assess the effects of chronic stress on the course of diabetes.

Relationship between personality and coping strategies and the course of diabetes.   Rovet and Ehrlich (1988) addressed the issue of temperament or personality and its possible effect on metabolic control in children with IDDM. Two standardized temperament questionnaires were completed by parents of 51 children with IDDM and 24 healthy control subjects. First, they observed no difference in temperament between diabetic children and sibling control subjects. There also was no unique diabetic temperament profile. However, using glycosylated hemoglobin as an outcome measure of metabolic control, they observed an effect of temperament on glycemic control. Diabetic children who were more active, were better at following routines, displayed milder responses to external stimuli, were less attentive, and were more prone to negative moods had improved metabolic control when compared with the other diabetic children. The authors avoided implying a cause-and-effect relationship. Because child and adolescent subjects may show marked variation in emotional maturity, in the extent of parental involvement and supervision, and in residual pancreatic ability to secrete insulin, these results cannot be generalized to other age groups. However, the study by Rovet and Ehrlich demonstrates the utility of developing methods of evaluation that are specific for the age group's psychological and medical characteristics.

A study by Stabler and colleagues (1987) also investigated the relationship between personality traits and glucose regulation in a psychophysiologic study of diabetic children. Children with Type A behavior, identified from their responses to video games, had a hyperglycemic response to stress that was not present in children with a Type B behavior pattern. In a study investigating the relationship between coping behavior and glucose control in diabetic adolescents, Delamater and colleagues (1987) found that those in poor control used significantly more wishful thinking and avoidance than those in better control. Hanson and colleagues (1987) found that the effects of stress on metabolic control in diabetic adolescents was buffered in subjects scoring high on measures of social competence; those with low social competence had marked worsening of metabolic control (as reflected in glycosylated hemoglobin) in response to stressful life events, and those with high social competence scores demonstrated minimal changes in metabolic control. Peyrot and McMurry (1992) reported that effective coping, defined as scoring below the median on a measure of "stress-dampening" coping styles and above the median for stress-exacerbating styles, protected individuals from the effects of stress on glycemic control. Kuttner and colleagues (1990) found the "learned helplessness" attributional style for negative events was significantly associated with glycosylated hemoglobin in a group of 50 diabetic children (10–16 years old). Learned helplessness was not associated with regimen adherence. Hanson and colleagues (1987) and Aikens and colleagues (1992) also found that stress had an effect on metabolic control that was independent of its effect on compliance.

Relationship between psychosocial interventions and the course of diabetes. Several studies have reported the effects of behavioral or psychosocial interventions on glucose control in diabetic patients. Surwit and Feinglos (1983) and Lammers and colleagues (1984) found that relaxation training can improve blood glucose control in non-IDDM diabetic patients. However, relaxation training has not produced consistent benefits in IDDM patients (Feinglos et al. 1987). Surwit and Feinglos (1988) speculated that stress may be of more importance in blood glucose fluctuations in non-IDDM than in IDDM patients. In their review, Helz and Templeton (1990) described several anecdotal reports that suggest that individual or family psychotherapy may improve diabetic control in some patients, but there are no controlled studies that demonstrate the efficacy of these interventions in enhancing diabetic control.

Summary

Although retrospective studies suggest a relationship between stressful life events and the course of diabetes mellitus, these studies are methodologically flawed. A well-controlled study of the effects of laboratory-induced stress on measures of glycemic control found there was no effect in both patients with diabetes mellitus and control subjects (Kemmer et al. 1986). However, laboratory studies, using within-subject designs, suggest that stress is associated with changes in glucose regulation in a subset of diabetic patients (Halford et al. 1990; Gonder-Frederick et al. 1990). Stress may also interact with dietary disinhibition to affect metabolic control (Balfour et al. 1993).

One prospective study (Lloyd et al. 1991) reported a relationship between stressful life events and the need for antihypertensive therapy. There is also some evidence to suggest that temperament and coping strategies influence glycemic control in diabetic children and adolescents (Delamater et al. 1987; Hanson et al. 1987; Kuttner et al. 1990; Rovet and Ehrlich 1988; Stabler et al. 1987) as well as adults (Peyrot and McMurry 1992). Relaxation training may improve blood glucose control in non-IDDM patients (Lammers et al. 1984; Surwit and Feinglos 1983), but there is no consistent benefit in IDDM patients (Feinglos et al. 1987). A review by Surwit and colleagues (1992) suggested that the influence of stress on metabolic control is moderated by the presence of autonomic neuropathy in IDDM patients. These authors also concluded that stress reliably produces hyperglycemia in non-IDDM, although this conclusion is based primarily on results from animal studies.

Graves' Disease

Since the first description of Graves' disease, otherwise known as exophthalmic goiter, clinicians have suspected that psychological and social factors contribute to its etiology and course (Weiner 1977). Graves' disease was one of the "holy seven" psychosomatic disorders studied by Alexander and described in his famous treatise, *Psychosomatic Medicine* (1950). Weiner's comprehensive and scholarly review of Alexander's work, as well as the work of more recent investigators who have studied the effects of psychological factors on Graves' disease, provide the basis for the discussion that follows.

It should be noted that almost all of the research studies that Weiner (1977) reviewed had serious methodological flaws, including retrospective or cross-sectional design, poorly defined patient populations, and lack of appropriate control groups. Also, the highly variable onset and course of Graves' disease makes it difficult to attribute changes in course to psychological and behavioral factors (Weiner 1977). Moreover, the hyperthyroid state that usually accompanies Graves' disease is itself characterized by a host of psychological, behavioral, and neuropsychiatric signs and symptoms (Hall et al. 1986; Loosen and Prange 1984; Wilson and Jefferson 1985). Because the early stages of Graves' disease may develop slowly, psychological and behavioral factors that appear to precede illness activity may actually be consequences of unrecognized changes in thyroid function (Weiner 1977). Weiner concluded from his extensive review of the literature that there is no evidence to suggest that psychological characteristics of patients predispose them to develop Graves' disease or any other thyroid disorder.

More recently, however, a population-based, case-controlled study was published that suggests negative life events may be risk factors for Graves' disease (Winsa et al. 1991). Over 2 years, 95% of 219 eligible patients with newly diagnosed Graves' disease and 372 matched control subjects answered an identical mailed questionnaire assessing demographic variables, life events, social support, and personality. Compared with control subjects, Graves' patients had more negative life events in the 12 months preceding the diagnosis; negative life-event scores were also significantly higher (odds ratio = 6.3) for the category with the highest negative score. Also, these investigators found that slightly more patients than control subjects were divorced. These results were independent of other possible confounding risk factors. Prospective studies are needed to confirm these findings. There is presently insufficient evidence to suggest that psychological factors affect the course of Graves' disease.

Cushing's Disease

Gifford and Gunderson (1970) reviewed the literature on the relationship between psychological factors and Cushing's disease and described 10 cases. They hypothesized that Cushing's disease represents a pathophysiological reaction to bereavement in predisposed individuals. Cushing argued that emotional stress contributed to the development of the disease that bears his name. He is quoted in Gifford and Gunderson's review: "Within normal physiological limits individuals differ greatly . . . in the character and degree of their secretory response under the influence of primitive emotions" (p. 171) and "under special psychic durance [these responses] may acquire a sufficient chronicity to lead to a so-called symptom-complex of disease" (p. 171) (Gifford and Gunderson 1970). However, most of the nonanimal studies that Gifford and Gunderson cited are retrospective, and no controlled studies in humans have been done, to our knowledge, that would either support or reject their hypothesis. Although stressful stimuli may acutely lead to increased secretion of corticosteroids, hypercortisolism cannot be equated with illness and disease. Moreover, hypercortisolism of several etiologies, including Cushing's disease, has been associated with the development of a wide range of neuropsychiatric phenomena (Hall et al. 1986). Thus, as Cushing also stated, there is "difficulty in determining which was the primary factor—the psychic instability or the disturbance of endocrine secretion" (Gifford and Gunderson 1970, p. 171).

Conclusions and Recommendations
for Further Research

There is a paucity of research on psychological factors affecting endocrine disorders, especially when considering endocrine disorders other than diabetes mellitus. Most of the studies that we surveyed were quite dated and had either a retrospective design or other serious methodological flaws. Diabetes mellitus appears to be the only endocrine disorder that has been the focus of recent research studies that are significantly improved in design. However, there have been no consistent results demonstrating that psychological factors affect the onset of diabetes mellitus. Only a small number of studies have demonstrated that psychological factors affect the course of diabetes, and most of these have reported the effects of acute stressors on measures of glucose control.

Several recommendations can be made for future research in this area. The methodology of studies in this area would be enhanced by prospective designs, well-defined subject populations, and meaningful control groups. There is a need to identify age-specific issues that might affect outcome; for example, children and adolescents with diabetes mellitus may react differently to a given stressor than adults. The use of better methods to measure long-term glycemic control (e.g., glycosylated hemoglobin) should help to assess the relationship between psychological factors and the course of diabetes mellitus. Laboratory paradigms to assess the physiological reactivity of the endocrine system to psychological challenges should be used and developed. These paradigms might help to elucidate further the psychophysiologic mechanisms that may underlie the relationships between psychological factors and endocrine diseases.

Psychological factors that have the most clinical relevance, such as anxiety and depression, should be investigated in prospective studies of patients with endocrine diseases. Creative ways to assess the impact of real-life stressors on endocrine function are also needed. Compliance with all aspects of the treatment or experimental intervention plan should always be monitored with both experimental and control subjects. Finally, there is an obvious need for well-designed research to study the effects of psychological factors on endocrine diseases other than diabetes mellitus.

References

Aikens JE, Wallander JL, Bell DS, et al: Daily stress variability, learned resourcefulness, regimen adherence, and metabolic control in type I diabetes mellitus: evaluation of a path model. J Consult Clin Psychol 60:113–118, 1992

Alexander F: Psychosomatic Medicine. New York, WW Norton, 1950

Balfour L, Romano White D, Schiffrin A, et al: Dietary disinhibition, perceived stress, and glucose control in young, type 1 diabetic women. Health Psychol 12:33–38, 1993

Cobb S, Rose RM: Hypertension, peptic ulcer and diabetes in air traffic controllers. JAMA 224:489–492, 1973

Delamater AM, Kurtz SM, Bubb J, et al: Stress and coping in relation to metabolic control of adolescents with type I diabetes. J Dev Behav Pediatr 8:136–140, 1987

Dunbar F: Psychosomatic Diagnosis. New York, PB Hoeber, 1943

Feinglos MN, Hastedt P, Surwit RS: Effects of relaxation therapy on patients with type I diabetes mellitus. Diabetes Care 10:72–75, 1987

Gendel BR, Benjamin JE: Psychogenic factors in the etiology of diabetes. N Engl J Med 234:556–560, 1946

Gifford S, Gunderson JG: Cushing's disease as a psychosomatic disorder: a selective review of the clinical and experimental literature and a report of ten cases. Perspect Biol Med 13:169–221, 1970

Goetsch VL: Stress and blood glucose in diabetes mellitus: a review and methodological commentary. Annals of Behavioral Medicine 11:102–107, 1989

Gonder-Frederick LA, Carter WR, Cox DJ, et al: Environmental stress and blood glucose change in IDDM. Health Psychol 9:503–515, 1990

Hagglof B, Blom L, Dahlquist G, et al: The Swedish childhood diabetes study: indications of severe psychological stress as a risk factor for type 1 (insulin-dependent) diabetes mellitus in childhood. Diabetologia 34:579–583, 1991

Halford WK, Cuddily S, Mortimer RH: Psychological stress and blood glucose regulation in type I diabetic patients. Health Psychol 9:516–528, 1990

Hall RCW, Stickney S, Beresford TP: Endocrine disease and behavior. Integrative Psychiatry 4:122–135, 1986

Hanson CL, Henggeler SW, Burghen GA: Social competence and parental support as mediators of the link between stress and metabolic control in adolescents with insulin-dependent diabetes mellitus. J Consult Clin Psychol 55:529–533, 1987

Helz JW, Templeton B: Evidence of the role of psychosocial factors in diabetes mellitus: a review. Am J Psychiatry 147:1275–1282, 1990

Hinkle LE Jr, Wolf S: The effects of stressful life situations on the concentration of blood glucose in diabetic and non-diabetic humans. Diabetes 1:383–392, 1952

Hinkle LE Jr, Conger GB, Wolf S: Studies on diabetes mellitus: the relation of stressful life situations to the concentration of ketone bodies in the blood of diabetic and non-diabetic humans. J Clin Invest 29:754–769, 1959

Kemmer FW, Bisping R, Steingruber HJ, et al: Psychological stress and metabolic control in patients with type I diabetes mellitus. N Engl J Med 314:1076–1084, 1986

Kuttner MJ, Delamater AM, Santiago JV: Learned helplessness in diabetic youths. J Pediatr Psychol 15:581–594, 1990

Lammers CA, Naliboff BD, Straatmeyer AJ: The effects of progressive relaxation on stress and diabetic control. Behav Res Ther 22:641–650, 1984

Lloyd CE, Robinson N, Stevens LK, et al: The relationship between stress and the development of diabetic complications. Diabetic Med 8:146–150, 1991

Loosen PT, Prange AJ Jr: Hormones of the thyroid axis and behavior, in Peptides, Hormones and Behavior. Edited by Nemeroff CB, Dunn AJ. New York, Spectrum Publications, 1984, pp 533–577

MacGillivray MH, Bruck E, Voorhess ML: Acute diabetic ketoacidosis in children: role of the stress hormones. Pediatr Res 15:99–106, 1981

Maudsley H: The Pathology of Mind, 3rd Edition. New York, Appleton, 1899

Menninger WC: Psychological factors in the aetiology of diabetes. J Nerv Ment Dis 81:1–13, 1935

Peyrot MF, McMurry J Jr: Stress buffering and glycemic control: the role of coping styles. Diabetes Care 15:842–846, 1992

Robinson N, Fuller JH: Role of life events and difficulties in the onset of diabetes mellitus. J Psychosom Res 29:583–591, 1985

Rovet J, Ehrlich RM: Effect of temperament on metabolic control in children with diabetes mellitus. Diabetes Care 11:77–82, 1988

Schless GL, von Laveran-Stiebar R: Recurrent episodes of diabetic acidosis precipitated by emotional stress. Diabetes 13:419–420, 1964

Stabler B, Surwit RS, Lane JD, et al: Type A behavior pattern and blood glucose control in diabetic children. Psychosom Med 49:313–316, 1987

Surwit RS, Feinglos MN: The effects of relaxation on glucose tolerance in non-insulin dependent diabetes. Diabetes Care 6:176–179, 1983

Surwit RS, Feinglos MN: Stress and autonomic nervous system in Type II diabetes: a hypothesis. Diabetes Care 11:83–85, 1988

Surwit RS, Schneider MS, Feinglos MN: Stress and diabetes mellitus. Diabetes Care 15:1413–1422, 1992

Vandenbergh RL, Sussman KE, Titus CC: Effects of hypnotically induced acute emotional stress on carbohydrate and lipid metabolism in patients with diabetes mellitus. Psychosom Med 28:382–390, 1966

Vandenbergh RL, Sussman KE, Vaughan GD: Effects of combined physical-anticipatory stress on carbohydrate-lipid metabolism in patients with diabetes mellitus. Psychosomatics 8:16–19, 1967

Weiner H: Psychobiology and Human Disease. New York, Elsevier, 1977

Willis T: Pharmaceutice rationalis, in The Works of Thomas Willis. London, England, Dring, Harper, & Leigh, 1684

Wilson WH, Jefferson JW: Thyroid disease, behavior, and psychopharmacology. Psychosomatics 26:481–492, 1985

Winsa B, Adami HO, Bergstrom R, et al: Stressful life events and Graves disease. Lancet 2:1475–1479, 1991

Psychological Factors Affecting Medical Conditions

Summary

ALAN STOUDEMIRE, M.D.

A s summarized by the literature reviews in this volume, evidence derived from case reports, case series, and systematic research studies has clearly demonstrated that psychological and behavioral factors may adversely affect the course of medical conditions in almost every major disease category, including diabetes (Beardsley and Goldstein 1993), dermatologic disorders (Folks and Kinney 1992a), gastrointestinal disorders (Folks and Kinney 1992b), cardiovascular disease (Goldstein and Niaura 1992; Niaura and Goldstein 1992), renal disease (Levenson and Glocheski 1991), oncological disease (Levenson and Bemis 1991), neurological conditions (McNamara 1991), and pulmonary and rheumatologic disorders (Moran 1991). In the following brief summary, I highlight a few examples of some of the findings from these literature surveys. Readers interested in more details are referred to the individual chapters of this text as well as several book chapters that have summarized in a concise fashion the essential findings of this project (McDaniel et al., in press; Stoudemire and McDaniel, in press; Stoudemire et al., in press).

The strongest association found between psychological factors and physical conditions was with depression (Wells et al. 1989). Depression has been associated with complicating the course of cerebrovascular stroke, multiple sclerosis, Parkinson's disease, and epilepsy (McNamara 1991). Depression also adversely affects the prognosis of myocardial infarction (Frasure-Smith et al. 1993; Goldstein and Niaura 1992) and renal disease (Levenson and Glocheski 1991). The presence of depression may affect the prognosis of certain cancers, probably through immunologic mechanisms (Levenson and Bemis 1991). High rates of depression have been observed with certain types of dermatologic conditions, specifically psoriasis and acne. Although dysphoric mood theoretically can affect adaptation to any illness, depression particularly has been noted to affect rehabilitative outcome in rheumatoid arthritis and stroke (Moran 1991). In general, increased rates of functional disability have been well documented in medical patients who are depressed (Carney et al. 1988; Wells et al. 1989).

Symptoms of anxiety and depression appear to be associated with the expression of disease symptoms (or to be associated with their perpetuation) in a variety of illnesses. Examples of conditions in which symptoms of anxiety and depression have been noted to affect the expression of illness include irritable bowel syndrome, esophageal motility disorders, peptic ulcer disease, Crohn's disease (regional enteritis), and acne.

Although a variety of personality traits have been associated with certain medical conditions (e.g., peptic ulcer disease, asthma, rheumatoid arthritis, inflammatory bowel disease, dermatoses), there has been no convincing evidence that any specific type of personality trait alone can account for the development of a particular physical illness, with the possible exception of coronary artery disease. The degree of adaptation to illness, particularly successful defenses against anxiety and the appropriate use of denial, actually may positively influence medical prognosis. Problematic personality traits of almost any type (including pathologic denial) can interfere with good working relationships with health care personnel and lead to behaviors that complicate the management of an illness.

The data regarding the relationship between heart disease and personality patterns that have received extensive attention nevertheless remain controversial. Evidence suggests, however, that patients exhibiting "Type A" (pressured, hostile) behavior, or its behavioral subcomponents, are at significantly greater risk for development of coronary artery disease. Other evidence indicates that anger and hostility may be the essential emotional subcomponents of the Type A behavior pattern involved in the pathogenesis of coronary artery disease. Data also indicate that chronic activation of the sympathetic nervous system during stressful behavioral challenges contributes to the development of atherosclerosis and vulnerability to cardiac arrhythmias. That sudden activation of the sympathetic nervous system under stressful conditions causes cardiac arrhythmias and occasionally sudden death is well established (Goldstein and Niaura 1992). Other cardiovascular conditions have been extensively studied with respect to psychological factors. Well-documented associations have been made in patients with preexisting coronary artery disease among stress reactions and myocardial ischemia and hypertensive responses.

Several other conditions in which stress responses associated with heightened physiologic reactivity lead to the expression or exacerbation of disease symptoms include urticarial reactions, eczema, atopic dermatitis, and pruritus. Exacerbations of asthmatic reactions in particular have been associated with stress reactions, although the mechanisms involved are not entirely clear (Folks and Kinney 1992a).

Although social and economic factors were not a specific focus of our literature reviews, it has also been well demonstrated that reduced levels of socioeconomic resources, social isolation, low social support, and employment that is both stressful and dissatisfying enhances risk for cardiovascular death from coronary artery disease after all other risk factors are controlled (Williams et al. 1992). Nonmarried individuals with coronary artery disease are also at higher risk for death compared with married individuals (Chandra et al. 1983; Wiklund et al. 1980).

Certain types of maladaptive health behavior, particularly cigarette smoking, overeating, and alcohol and drug use, have a major impact on public health. These health behaviors compose the preponderance of potentially preventable medical morbidity and mortality in the United States (Stoudemire and Hales 1991; Stoudemire et al. 1986). Alcohol and substance abuse and dependence, including nicotine abuse and dependence, have been recognized as adversely affecting health and medical conditions. (Cigarette smoking [nicotine dependence], alcohol, and other substances, however, are not included under "psychological factors affecting medical conditions" because these problems are covered in separate diagnostic categories in DSM-IV [American Psychiatric Association 1994].)

The fact that psychological factors and psychiatric disorders may affect the clinical course of medical illness is now incontrovertible and is no longer a topic of serious debate. What is less understood, however, is why certain individual patients appear to be more vulnerable to such deleterious effects, particularly in respect to the role of genetic risk factors. The critical research agenda for the next decade, however, is in developing the kinds of prevention interventions that enhance psychological resilience to medical illnesses and the extent that early and timely detection and treatment of psychiatric illness in the context of medical illness would improve outcome. As has been discussed in this volume, research has already established that survival is improved after interventions to enhance the patient's ability to cope and to deal with emotional distress following treatment for both breast cancer and malignant melanoma (Fawzy et al. 1993; Spiegel et al. 1989). Similar interventions are needed in other disease categories, such as in myocardial infarction, to establish the effectiveness of psychiatric therapies in improving medical outcomes. Further demonstration of the practical effectiveness of treating psychiatric complications of medical illness, including prevention strategies, will greatly enhance the acceptance of psychiatry in mainstream medicine. Hence, the ensuing years will likely be promising for increased involvement of psychiatry in medicine, as more scientific research validates the effectiveness of behavioral prevention strategies and psychiatric interventions in improving the prognosis of medical conditions.

Despite the complexities in ascertaining the precise associations between psychological factors and medical conditions, a reasonable amount of empirically based evidence now clearly exists to affirm unequivocally that psychological factors affect the course of most medical conditions. It is hoped that this series of reviews consolidating the literature on the relationship between psychological factors and medical conditions, and the development of more refined diagnostic criteria in DSM-IV to denote such interactions, will facilitate improved recognition of such relationships and assist in better patient care.

References

American Psychiatric Association: Diagnostic and Statistical Manual of Mental Disorders, 4th Edition. Washington, DC, American Psychiatric Association, 1994

Beardsley G, Goldstein MG: Psychological factors affecting physical condition: endocrine disease literature review. Psychosomatics 34:12–19, 1993

Carney RM, Rich MW, Freedland KE, et al: Major depressive disorder predicts cardiac events in patients with coronary artery disease. Psychosom Med 50:627–633, 1988

Chandra V, Szklo M, Goldberg R, et al: The impact of marital status on survival after an acute myocardial infarction: a population-based study. Am J Epidemiol 117:320–325, 1983

Fawzy FI, Fawzy NW, Hyun CS, et al: Malignant melanoma: effects of an early structured psychiatric intervention, coping, and affective state on recurrence and survival 6 years later. Arch Gen Psychiatry 50:681–689, 1993

Folks DG, Kinney FC: The role of psychological factors in dermatologic conditions. Psychosomatics 33:45–54, 1992a

Folks DG, Kinney FC: The role of psychological factors in gastrointestinal conditions: a review pertinent to DSM-IV. Psychosomatics 33:257–270, 1992b

Frasure-Smith N, Lesperance F, Talajic M: Depression following myocardial infarction: impact on 6-month survival. JAMA 270:1819–1825, 1993

Goldstein MG, Niaura R: Psychological factors affecting physical condition: cardiovascular disease literature review, part 1: coronary artery disease and sudden death. Psychosomatics 33:134–145, 1992

Levenson JL, Bemis C: The role of psychological factors in cancer onset and progression. Psychosomatics 32:124–132, 1991

Levenson JL, Glocheski S: Psychological factors affecting end-stage renal disease: a review. Psychosomatics 32:382–389, 1991

McDaniel JS, Moran MG, Levenson JL, et al: Psychological factors affecting medical conditions, in American Psychiatric Press Textbook of Psychiatry, 2nd Edition. Edited by Hales RE, Yudofsky SC, Talbott JA. Washington, DC, American Psychiatric Press, 1994, pp 565–590

McNamara ME: Psychological factors affecting neurological conditions: depression and stroke, multiple sclerosis, Parkinson's disease, and epilepsy. Psychosomatics 32:255–267, 1991

Moran MG: Psychological factors affecting pulmonary and rheumatologic diseases. Psychosomatics 32:14–23, 1991

Niaura R, Goldstein MG: Psychological factors affecting physical condition: cardiovascular disease literature review, part 2: coronary artery disease and sudden death and hypertension. Psychosomatics 33:146–155, 1992

Spiegel DS, Kraemer HC, Bloom JR, et al: Effect of a psychosocial treatment on survival of patients with metastatic breast cancer. Lancet 2:888–891, 1989

Stoudemire A, Hales RE: Psychological and behavioral factors affecting medical conditions and DSM-IV: an overview. Psychosomatics 32:5–13, 1991

Stoudemire A, McDaniel JS: History and current trends in psychosomatic medicine, in Comprehensive Textbook of Psychiatry, 6th Edition. Edited by Kaplan HI, Sadock BJ. Baltimore, MD, Williams & Wilkins (in press)

Stoudemire A, Frank R, Hedemark N, et al: The economic burden of depression. Gen Hosp Psychiatry 8:387–394, 1986

Stoudemire A, Beardsley G, Folks DG, et al: Psychological factors affecting physical condition (PFAPC) 316.00: proposals for revisions in DSM-IV, in DSM-IV Sourcebook, Vol 2. Edited by Widiger TA, Frances A, Pincus H, et al. Washington, DC, American Psychiatric Association (in press)

Wells KB, Stewart A, Hays RD, et al: The functioning and well-being of depressed patients. JAMA 262:914–919, 1989

Wiklund I, Oden A, Sanne H, et al: Prognostic importance of somatic and psychosocial variables after a first myocardial infarction. Am J Epidemiol 128:786–795, 1980

Williams RB, Barefoot JC, Califf RM, et al: Prognostic importance of social and economic resources among medically treated patients with angiographically documented coronary artery disease. JAMA 267:520–524, 1992

Index

*Page numbers printed in **boldface** type refer to tables and figures.*